CAMBRIDGE LIBRARY COLLECTION

Books of enduring scholarly value

Perspectives from the Royal Asiatic Society

A long-standing European fascination with Asia, from the Middle East to China and Japan, came more sharply into focus during the early modern period, as voyages of exploration gave rise to commercial enterprises such as the East India companies, and their attendant colonial activities. This series is a collaborative venture between the Cambridge Library Collection and the Royal Asiatic Society of Great Britain and Ireland, founded in 1823. The series reissues works from the Royal Asiatic Society's extensive library of rare books and sponsored publications that shed light on eighteenth- and nineteenth-century European responses to the cultures of the Middle East and Asia. The selection covers Asian languages, literature, religions, philosophy, historiography, law, mathematics and science, as studied and translated by Europeans and presented for Western readers.

Ulfáz Udwiyeh, or the Materia Medica

This materia medica – a book of collected knowledge about medicines and their properties – was originally written in Persian by Noureddeen Mohammed Abdullah al-Shirazi (fl.1625–40), physician to the Mughal emperor Shah Jahan, to whom it was dedicated. This 1793 publication contains entries in Persian, Arabic and Hindi, with English translations by Francis Gladwin (1744–1812), an employee of the East India Company and professor of Persian at Fort William College. The work begins by giving traditional Arabic evaluations of each type of medicine in terms of its power on a scale of 1 to 4, before presenting the dictionary of over 1,400 medicines, some with notes on their properties and usage. Providing an insight into healing practices in India in the seventeenth and eighteenth centuries, this work remains of interest to scholars in the history of medicine.

Cambridge University Press has long been a pioneer in the reissuing of out-of-print titles from its own backlist, producing digital reprints of books that are still sought after by scholars and students but could not be reprinted economically using traditional technology. The Cambridge Library Collection extends this activity to a wider range of books which are still of importance to researchers and professionals, either for the source material they contain, or as landmarks in the history of their academic discipline.

Drawing from the world-renowned collections in the Cambridge University Library and other partner libraries, and guided by the advice of experts in each subject area, Cambridge University Press is using state-of-the-art scanning machines in its own Printing House to capture the content of each book selected for inclusion. The files are processed to give a consistently clear, crisp image, and the books finished to the high quality standard for which the Press is recognised around the world. The latest print-on-demand technology ensures that the books will remain available indefinitely, and that orders for single or multiple copies can quickly be supplied.

The Cambridge Library Collection brings back to life books of enduring scholarly value (including out-of-copyright works originally issued by other publishers) across a wide range of disciplines in the humanities and social sciences and in science and technology.

Ulfáz Udwiyeh

or the Materia Medica

In the Arabic, Persian, and Hindevy Languages

NOUREDDEEN MOHAMMED ABDULLAH AL-SHIRAZI
TRANSLATED BY FRANCIS GLADWIN

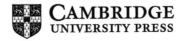

CAMBRIDGE
UNIVERSITY PRESS

CAMBRIDGE UNIVERSITY PRESS

Cambridge, New York, Melbourne, Madrid, Cape Town,
Singapore, São Paolo, Delhi, Mexico City

Published in the United States of America by Cambridge University Press, New York

www.cambridge.org
Information on this title: www.cambridge.org/9781108056090

© in this compilation Cambridge University Press 2013

This edition first published 1793
This digitally printed version 2013

ISBN 978-1-108-05609-0 Paperback

الغاظ ادویه
تصنیف نورالدین محمد عبدالله شیرازی

ULFAZ UDWIYEH,

OR THE

MATERIA MEDICA,

IN THE

Arabic, Persian, and Hindevy Languages.

COMPILED BY

NOUREDDEEN MOHAMMED ABDULLAH SHIRÁZY,

PHYSICIAN TO THE EMPEROR SHÁHJEHÁN.

WITH AN ENGLISH TRANSLATION,
BY
FRANCIS GLADWIN.

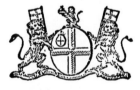

CALCUTTA:
PRINTED AT THE CHRONICLE PRESS.
MDCCXCIII.

JOHN LAIRD, Esq.

PRESIDENT, AND MEMBERS

OF THE HOSPITAL BOARD,

FORT WILLIAM.

GENTLEMEN,

THE following Work being publiſhed at your Recommendation, for the uſe of the Honourable Company, I beg leave to place it under your immediate Protection.

I HAVE THE HONOUR TO BE,

GENTLEMEN,

YOUR MOST OBEDIENT,

HUMBLE SERVANT,

FRANCIS GLADWIN.

CALCUTTA,
SEPTEMBER 10, 1793.

INTRODUCTION.

OF MEDICINES IN GENERAL.

THE Arabian phyficians, in defcribing the quality or power of medicines, make ufe of four degrees.

The FIRST DEGREE, is that whofe quality makes imperceptible impreffion; fuch as thofe that are hot; or thofe that are cold, &c. but which are not felt, unlefs they are reiterated. The SECOND DEGREE, is that which is more powerful than the former, but not fo much as to occafion any vifible injury. The THIRD DEGREE is that whofe impreffion is effentially hurtful, but not fo as to deftroy. The FOURTH DEGREE, is that whofe nature is fuch that it either kills or materially injures; and this is the property of poifonous medicines.

NAMES.	HOT.	COLD.	DRY.	MOIST.
	DEGREES.			
افسنتين *ÁFSUNTEEN* Wormwood	1	0	3	0
بابونه *Bá-bo/neh* Camomile flowers	1	0	1	0
تمر *Temr* Date	1	0	0	0
تخم كتان *Tokhem kut-án* Linfeed	1	0	0	0
حمّص *Himmis* A fpecies of vetch	1	0	3	1
رمان *Rum-mán* Pomegranate	1	0	0	0
حلزون *Hulzoon* Snail	1	0	0	0
شاهترة *Sháhtereh* Fumitory	1	0	2	0
صبر *Syb-ir* Aloes	1	0	3	0
لوف *Loof* Dragonwort	1	0	0	0
لادن *Làdun* Labdanum	1	0	0	0

B

اسقاقس

NAMES.	QUALITIES.			
	HOT.	COLD.	DRY.	MOIST.
	DEGREES.			
استقاتس *Iſka-kiſs* A ſpecies of melilot	2	o	o	o
اصل الغرب *Aſſul ul ghur-eb* Root of the mountain pine	2	o	o	o
اصل المازريون *Aſſul ul mázreeyoon* Mezereon root	2	o	3	o
سپيد وسياه بادروج *Sepeid wu ſeyáh badrooj*, Two ſpecies of ſweet baſil	2	o	o	o
برنجاسف *Bir-en-já-ſif* Mugwort	2	o	o	o
بلسان *Bulſán* The balſam tree	2	o	2	o
بزر الانجره *Buz-ir-ul-unjereh* Nettle ſeed, alſo the leaves, an infuſion of	2	o	o	o
جندبيدستر *Joondbeyduſter* Caſtor	2	o	2	o
حلبه *Hulbeh* Fenugreek	2	o	o	o
دبق *Dibk* A ſmall grain which is very viſcous	2	o	o	o
درديعصاره زيتون *Doordee aſſáreh zietoon* Dregs of olive oil	2	o	3	o
زراوندطويل ومدحرج *Zeráwund teweel wu Moodehrej* Birthwort, long, and round	2	o	2	o
زعفران *Zá-frán* Saffron	2	o	o	o
شبت *Shib-it* Fennel	2	o	o	o
عسل *Aſſul* Honey	2	o	2	o
عنصل *Unſul* Squill	2	o	o	o

NAMES.		QUALITIES.			
		HOT.	COLD.	DRY.	MOIST.
			DEGREES.		
قثاءالحمار	*Kiſſa-ul-hymár* Wild cucumber	2	0	0	0
فراسيون	*Frd-ſee-yoon* Euphraſia, eyebright	2	0	0	0
قشورشجرة الحية	*Kuſhoor, ſhijuret ul hyut* Gentian bark	2	0	0	0
قصب الزريرة	*Kuſſeb us ze-ree-ráh* Wormwood plant.	2	0	2	0
كبريت	*Kib-reet* Sulphur	2	0	0	0
كرفس	*Kerefs* Parſley	2	0	0	0
كمافيطوس	*Kum-d-fec-toos* Ground pine	2	0	3	0
كندر	*Koondir* Frankincenſe, of which there are three kinds	2	0	1	0
مصطكي	*Moos-te-ká* Maſtich	2	0	2	0
ملح	*Mil-h* Culinary ſalt	2	0	0	0
ميعه	*Mee-áh* Storax	2	0	0	0
وسخ الكوارير	*Wuſk-ul-ke-wá-reer* Freſh bees' wax	2	0	0	0
انيسون	*Ance-ſoon* Aniſeed	3	0	3	0
اسارون	*Aſſi-roon* Aſarabaca	3	0	3	0
افتيمون	*Afteemoon* Dodder of thyme	3	0	3	0
فنجنكشت	*Funj-ungooſht* Agnus caſtus, or the chaſte tree, it's leaves and ſeed	3	0	3	0
پودنهجبلي	*Pode-neh Je-be-lee* Wild mint	3	0	0	0
ترب	*Toorb* Radiſh, the root, and alſo the leaves	3	0	2	0
جاوشير	*Ji-we-ſheer* Gum opopanax	2	0	2	0

حاشا

NAMES.	QUALITIES.			
	HOT.	COLD.	DRY.	MOIST.
	DEGREES.			
حاشا *Há-ſhá* thyme	3	0	3	0
حرمل *Hirmul* Seed of wild rue	3	0	0	0
حاما *He-má-má* True amomum	3	0	0	0
خربقين *Khir-be-kine* The two hellebores	3	0	0	0
سداب *Sozd-áb* Rue	3	0	3	0
سرو *Sir-ou* The cypreſs tree	3	0	4	0
سكبينج *Suck-bee-nej* Gum ſagapenum	3	0	0	0
سلينخه *Se-lee-kheh* Caſſia lignea	3	0	3	0
شب محرق *Shelb-moh-ruck* Burnt alum	3	0	3	0
شراب كهنه *She-ráb kohneh* Old wine	3	0	3	0
شعر محرق *Sheir moh-ruck* Burnt hair	3	0	3	0
شيح ارمني محرق *Sheeh urmenee mohruck* A ſpecies of wormſeed burnt	3	0	3	0
صوف محرق *Soof moh-ruck* Burnt wool	3	0	0	0
غار *Ghár* Laurel	3	0	3	0
فوذنج نهري *Fode-nej neh-ree* Water mint	3	0	3	0
قشور قصب محرق *Kuſhoor kuſſeb moh-ruck* Burnt bark of the reed	3	0	3	0
قنه *Koon-neh* Galbanum	3	0	0	0
كرويا *Koor-weeya* Caraway ſeed	3	0	3	0
كاشم *Kúſhim* Lovage	3	0	0	0

كرفس بري

NAMES.			QUALITIES.		
		HOT.	COLD.	DRY.	MOIST.
			DEGREES.		
كرفس بري	*Ke-refs bir-ree* Wild parfley	3	o	o	o
كمادريوس	*Ke-má-der-yoos* Germander	3	o	3	o
مرماحوز	*Mir-má-hooz* An odoriferous plant	3	o	o	o
مرزنجوش	*Mir-zun-joofh* Marjoram	3	o	3	o
نانخواه	*Nán-kháwh* Bifhop's weed, ammi	3	o	o	o
نعناع	*Ná-ná-á* A fpecies of mint, very pungent	3	o	o	o
ينبوت	*Yum-boct* An Arabian pulfe	3	o	3	o
وج	*Waj* fweet flag	3	o	3	o
يتوعات	*Ye-too-dát* General name for milky plants	3	o	o	o
بصل	*Be-fel* Onion	4	o	o	o
ثوم	*Soom* Garlic	4	o	4	o
زيد البحر	*Ze-bed'ul behr* Foam of the fea, that adheres to rocks	4	o	o	o
سداب بري	*Soo-dáb bir-ree* Wild rue	4	o	o	o
فربيون	*Fir-be-yoon* Euphorbium	4	o	o	o
قسط	*Kouft* Coftus	4	o	o	o
قطران	*Kit-rán* Pitch	4	o	4	o
كراث	*Koor-ráfs* Leek	4	o	4	o
اصل السوس	*Uffu'lus' foos* Liquorice root	o	I	I	o
اقاقيانا شسته	*A'ka-kyá ná fhoof-teh* Acacia not wafhed, or prepared	o	I	3	o
برك قصب	*Birg kuffeb* Leaves of the reed	o	o	o	o
براده نحاس	*Boo-ra-deh no-háfs* Copper filings	o	o	o	o

C

برك بنفشه

NAMES.		QUALITIES.			
		HOT.	COLD.	DRY.	MOIST.
			DEGREES.		
برک بنغشه	*Birg be-nuf-sheh* Violet leaves	o	1	o	o
بسفايج	*Buss-fá-yej* Polypody	o	1	3	o
بلوط	*Bu-loot* Acorn	o	1	3	o
ثمرةالعليق	*Sumrétul u-leik* Blackberry	o	1	o	o
ثيل	*Seel* Couch grafs	o	1	o	o
جاورس	*Ja-wirfs* A fpecies of millet	o	1	o	o
جبن‌رطب	*Jubn-retb* New cheefe	o	1	o	o
خشخاش	*Khufh-kháfh* Poppy	o	1	o	o
دلب	*Doolb* The plane tree	o	1·	o	o
دهن‌الورد	*Duhn ul wurd* Oil of rofes	o	1	o	1
زجاج	*Zoojáj* Glafs	o	1	o	o
زنجفر	*Zunjefr* Cinnabar, native	o	1	o	o
سرمق	*Sir-muck* Stinking orach	o	1	o	2
شجرةالنبق	*Shejrut'n-nubk* The lote tree	o	1	o	o
عجم‌الزبيب	*Ujm uz zebeeb* Grape ftones	o	1	2	o
كمثري	*Koomnufra'* Pear	o	1	1	o
ماميثا	*Má-my-fá* The expreffed juice of a fpecies of poppy	o	1	o	o
نشاسته	*Na-fháf-teh* Starch	o	1	o	o
هندبا	*Hindbá* Endive	o	1	o	o
اقاقيامغسول	*Akd-ky-á mugh-foil* Wafhed (prepared) acacia	o	2	o	o
اطراف‌وبرک زيتون	*Utráf wu berg zietoon* Leaves and branches of the olive tree	o	2	3	o

هليون

NAMES.	QUALITIES.			
	HOT.	COLD.	DRY.	MOIST.
		DEGREES.		
هليون *Hil-yoon* Afparagus	o	2	o	o
بطيخ *Beteek.* Mufk melon	o	2	o	2
يمانيه *Yema-nee-a* A fpecies of chicory, growing in marfhy places	o	2	o	2
بزرقطونا *Buz-ir ke-too-na* Fleawort feed	o	2	o	o
جبار *Jummár* Pith of the date tree	o	2	o	o
خوخ *Khoakh* Peach	o	2	o	I
خيار *Khyár* Cucumber	o	2	o	I
رصاص *Réffáfs* Tin	o	2	o	o
زيتون خام *Zietoon khám* Unripe olives	o	2	o	o
سماق *Sumák* Sumach	o	2	o	o
تخم اترج *Tokhum ootruj* Citron feed	o	2	o	o
طحلب *Tuh-leb* Water mofs	o	2	o	I
عفص *Uf-ifs* Gall apple, unripe	o	2	o	o
كدو *Ké-doo* A large kind of cucumber, or gourd, with a thin rind	o	2	o	o
لسان الحمل *Leffán ul huml* Narrow-leav'd plantain, or ribwort	o	2	4	o
ماش *Máfh* A fmall kind of grain	o	2	o	o
مغرة *Moghreh* Red earth	o	2	o	o
كلم *Ke-lum* Cabbage	o	2	2	o
برشيان دارو *Bir-fhe-an-da-roo* A pot-herb of a red colour	o	2	o	o
بقلةالحمقا *Bucklet'l humeká* Purflain	o	2	o	2

جلنار

NAMES.		QUALITIES.			
		HOT.	COLD.	DRY.	MOIST.
			DEGREES.		
جلنار	*Joolnar* Wild rofe	o	3	3	o
حب العليق خام	*Hub ul uleik kham* Unripe blackberries	o	3	3	o
حماض الاترج	*Hum-áz-ul ooturj* Citron jui	o	3	o	o
حي العالم	*Hy-ul-aálum* Houfe-leek	o	3	1	o
خشخاش سياه	*Khufh-káfh fee-áh* Black poppy	o	3	o	o
عصي الراعي	*Afyr'rá-ey* A pot-herb of a red colour	o	3	o	o
لفاح	*Loo-fáh* Fruit of the mandrake	o	3	o	o
افيون	*Af-yoon* Opium	o	4	o	o
شوكران	*Showkran* Hemlock	o	4	o	o
لبن خشخاش	*Lebn Khufhkhafh* Milk of the poppy	o	4	o	o
اصل النيل	*Uffel ul neel* Root of the *neel* tree	o	o	1	o
بادام شيرين	*Bádám fhereen* Sweet almond	o	o	1	o
پرسياوشان	*Pir-fy-ow-fhán* Maiden hair	o	o	1	o
پوست جوز	*Poaft jowz* Walnut fhells	o	o	1	o
تخم خربزه	*Tokhem Khirboozéh* Mufk melon feed	o	o	1	o
حب الغار	*Hub ul ghár* Laurel berries	o	o	1	o
اب انجره	*Ab Unjereh* Juice of nettles	o	o	1	o
حزاز الصخر	*Huzáz uf fuckher* Mofs that grows on ftones, &c.	o	o	1	o
دفلي	*Diflee* Rhododaphne	o	o	1	o
رازيانه	*Rázee-áneh* A fpecies of anifeed	o	o	1	o
روغن جوز	*Rughen jowz* Oil of walnuts	o	o	1	o
زعفران	*Za-frán* Saffron	o	o	1	o

سويق الشعر

NAMES.	QUALITIES.			
	HOT.	COLD.	DRY.	MOIST.
			DEGREES.	
سعد *Sáád* A prickly plant, of which camels are very fond	o	o	I	o
سويق الشعير *Seweek us shy-eer* Wheat flour	o	o	o	o
صعتر *Sá tur* Origanum, or wild marjoram	o	o	I	o
صبغ جوز *Semugh jowz* Walnut-tree gum	o	o	I	o
ورق سوسن *Weruck So-sun* Lily leaves	o	o	I	o
اصل المر *Uſſul ul murr* Root of the myrrh tree	o	o	2	o
اصل اللوف *Uſſul ul loof* Root of dragonwort	o	o	2	o
بيخ نيلوفر *Beykh neeloofir* Root of the water lily	o	o	2	o
حبة الخضرا *Hubbet-'ul khuzra* Juniper berries	3	o	2	o
زفت *Ziſt* Pitch	o	o	2	o
سنبل الطيب *Sembel ut' teib* Spikenard	o	o	2	o
سنبل رومي *Sembel roomee* Celtic nard	o	o	2	o
شجرة مصطكي *Shejereh muſtekí* The maſtich tree	o	o	2	o
قفر اليهود *Kufr-ul yehood* Jew's pitch	o	o	2	o
شيلم *Sheelum* Tares	2	o	2	o
قشور الاترج *Ke-ſhoor-ul-oot-ruj* Citron peel	o	o	2	o
كرنب *Kirnub* Cabbage	o	o	2	o
كرسنه *Kur-ſeneh* Pea	o	o	2	o
لبن *Lebn* Milk	o	o	2	o
مر مكي *Murr muck-kee* Mecca myrrh	o	o	3	o
نسيج العنكبوة *Nesj-ul-unkeboot* Cobweb	o	o	2	o
ابهل *Ub-hel* Seed of the mountain pine	o	o	3	o
اصل فنطافلون *Uſſul fenta-fe-loon* Root of cinquefoil	o	o	3	o

D

كرنب خشك

NAMES.	QUALITIES.			
	HOT.	COLD.	DRY.	MOIST.
		DEGREES.		
كرنب‌خشك *Kirnub Kooſkh* Dried cabbage	o	o	3	o
بوره *Booráh* Borax	o	o	3	o
پوست‌غرب سوخته *Poaſt gherb Sokkteh* Bark of the mountain pine, burnt	o	o	3	o
حلتيت *Hil teeí* Aſafœtida	o	o	3	o
حماض الاترج *Hum-az ul Ootruj* Citron juice	o	o	3	o
دارشيشعان *Dár-ſhe-ſháen* An aromatic bark of a prickly tree	o	o	3	o
دخن *Dukhen* A kind of grain reſembling millet	o	o	3	o
زباد *Ze'bad* Civet	o	o	3	o
رماد‌حلزون بري *Ré-mád hulzoon bir-ree* Calcined wood-ſnails	o	o	3	I
روغن‌ترب *Roghen toorb* Oil of radiſh	o	o	3	o
زوفا *Zoofá* Hyſſop	o	o	3	o
سداب‌بوستاني *Soodáb boſtánee* Garden rue	o	o	3	2
سرطان‌محرق *Sirtán Mohruck* Calcined crabs	o	o	3	o
سركه *Seer-keh* Vinegar	o	o	3	o
شب‌محرق *Shub mohruck* Burnt alum	o	o	3	o
شونيز *Shoo-neez*, commonly called *See-ah daneh*, or black feed	o	o	3	o
وف‌محرق *Soof mohruck* Burnt wool	o	o	3	o
فاوانيا *Fá-dá-nyá* A root reſembling the carrot	o	o	3	o

فاشرا

NAMES.		QUALITIES.			
		HOT.	COLD.	DRY.	MOIST.
				DEGREES.	
فاشرا Fá-she-rá Briony		o	o	3	o
فطراساليون Fit-ra-sá-li-yoon Parsley		o	o	3	o
قيصوم Ky-soom Southernweed		o	o	3	o
كرفس بري Kerfs bir-ree Wild parsley		o	o	3	o
مشكطرا مشبع Misk-kee-tara-meshugh Dittany of Crete		o	o	3	o
ورق غار Werek ghár Laurel leaves		o	o	3	o
خردل Khirdul Mustard seed		o	o	4	o
كرم Kerm Vine branches		o	o	4	o
برك بنفشه Berg-bé-nuf-sheh Violet leaves		o	o	o	1
خصية الثعلب Khuseyet us sáleb Satyrion		o	o	o	1
عصاره سوسن U-sa-reh so-sun Expressed juice of lillies		o	o	o	1
كاهو Kd-hoo Lettuce		o	o	o	1
لسان الثور Lissán us sáur Ox tongue, buglofs		o	o	o	1
قرع Kurá Gourd with thin rind		o	o	o	2
مشمش Mishmish Apricot		o	o	o	2
دم الاخوين Dum ul ákhwein Dragon's blood		o	o	o	1
شجر جوز Shejir jowz Walnut tree		o	o	o	1
فطر Fithr Mushroom		o	o	o	1
ورق عليق Werek Uleik Bramble leaves		o	2	o	1
اصل الخنثي Ussul ul khunsá The hermaphrodite root		1	1	o	o
حب الصنوبر Hnb us sonobur Pine kernels		1	1	o	o
خربزة Khirboozeh Musk melon		1	1	o	o
زيت Ziet Olive oil		1	1	o	o
زيتون Zietoon Olives		1	1	o	o

سرخس

NAMES.	QUALITIES.			
	HOT.	COLD.	DRY.	MOIST.
	DEGREES.			
سرخس Sir-ukhs Root of spleenwort, mule's fern	I	2	0	0
شمع Shum-a Bees' wax	I	I	0	0
طين ساموس Teen samoos Samian earth	I	I	0	0
مرداسنك Murdarsung Litharge of lead	I	I	0	0

مخدرات MOKEDERRÁT.——NARCOTICA.

اذاراقي Uzá-rá-kee Seed of a poison-ous Indian root

اسپند Is-pund Wild rue

اصل الذرة Ussel uz zooret Root of a spe-cies of grain, commonly called jáwirs

اصل اللغاح Ussel ul Loofah Mandrake root

افيون Uf yoon Opium

بيخ موته جنكلي Beykh mowteh junglee Root of a species of grass

تخم وبرك تنباكو Tokhem wu berg tumbákoo Seed and leaves of tobacco

جوز ماثل Jowz má.fil The thorn apple

سراج القطرب Sē-ráj-ul kootreb The fairy's lamp: a plant which shines at night like the glow-worm

شبيبي She-bee-bee A narotic root

شوكران Shukrán Hemlock

قنب Kinnub Hemp

كاكنج Káknej Winter cherry

لبن الخيل Lebn ul ki·el Mare's milk

لونك جنكلي Lowng junglee Wild cloves

مسهلات صفرا MOOS-HIL-ÁT SUF-RÁ.——CHOLAGOGA.

اجاص Ij jáfs A species of plum

افستين Afsunteen Wormwood

بنفشه خشك Beneffhch Khoofkh Dried violets

ترنجبين Tu-renjebeen A species of manna

تمر هندي Temr-hindee Tamarind

خيار شنبر Khy-ar-fhumber Caffia fiftu-laris

سقمونيا Suc-mo-nya Scammony

شاهتره Shah-tereh Fumitory

شبرم

شبرم *Shibrum* A species of spurge

شیرخشت *Sheer-khisht* Manna

صبر *S b ir* Aloes

کلسرخ *Gool soorkh* Red roses

لبلاب *Lublâb* Ivy

مازریون *Mâz-ri-yoon* Mezereon

هليلهزرد { *He-ley-leh zird* Yellow myrobolans.

مسهلات بلغم *MOOS HIL-AT BELGHEM.*——PHLEGMAGOGA.

بسفايج *Bis-fâ-ij* Polypody

تربد *Toorbood* Turbith root

حب النيل { *Hub ul neel* Berries of a blue creeper

حرمل *Hirmul* Wild rue

شحم حنظل { *Shēm henzil* Pulp of colo-quintida

غاريقون *Ghâ-r e-koon* Agaric

فرفيون *Fir-fee-yoon* Euphorbium

قثاءالحمار *Kiffâ ul hymar* Wild cucumber

قنطوريون *Kun-too-reeyoon* Centaury

ماهيزهرج { *Mâhee-zeh-ruj* A species of creeper

ماهودانه { *Mâhoo-dáneh* A small red seed called also *hub ul mullook ·*

مسهلات سودا *MOOS-HIL-ÁT SOWDÁ.*——MELANAGOGA.

افتيمون *Aftcemoon* Dodder of thyme

اسطوخودوس { *Us-too-khoo-doos* Stoechas, French lavender

امله *Á. mu-leh* Emblic myrobolans

بالنكو { *Bâ-lun-goo* A species of sweet bafil

بسفايج *Bisfâ-ij* Polypody

حجرلاجورد *Hejr lâ'j-wird* Lapis lazuli

سنا *Sē-nâ* Senna

غاريقون *Ghâ-ree-koon* Agaric

كشوث *Koo-fhoos* The herb curfuta

هليلهكابلي { *He-ley-leh câbulee* Chebuli myrobolans

مقيبات *MOKI YE-ÁT.*——EMETICA.

اب كدوي تلخ { *Áb kud-oo telkh* Juice of bitter gourd

بورة *Boorah* Borax

تخم وبرك ترب { *Tokhem wu birg toorb* Seed and leaves of radish

تخم شبت *Tokhem Sheb-it* Fennel seed

تخم جرجير

E

تخم‌جرجير	*Tokhem-jir-jeer* Seed of wild rocket
تخم‌مازريون	*Tokhem máz-ri-yoon* Seed of wild spurge
خربق	*Khir-buc* Hellebore
سكنجبين	*Sĕ-ken-je-been* Oxymel of vinegar and honey
كنكرزد	*Kunkir zud* Artichoke gum

كندش	*Koondoosh* Glasswort
لوبيای‌سرخ	*Loo-beeyá Soorkh* A red pot-herb
ماءالعسل	*Má ul ássel* Water and honey
موبزج	*Mĕ-wee-zuj* Raisins
نمك‌هندي	*Ne-muck hindee* Salt of bitumen.

مفتحات   MU-FE'TTÉ-HÁT.——DEOBSTRUENTIA.

اذخر	*Iz-keir* Camel's hay
اسطوخودوس	*Us-too-koo-doos* Stoechas
افتيمون	*Afteemoon* Dodder of thyme
افسنتين	*Áfsunteen* Wormwood
انيسون	*Á-nee-soon* Aniseed
ايرسا	*Iyr-sa* Root of blue Iris
ترمس	*Toormiss* Egyptian lupin
جنطيانا	*Gen-ti-á-ná* Gentian
حاشا	*Há-shá* Thyme
حرمل	*Hirmul* Wild rue
حماما	*Hĕ-má-má* Amomum
دارچيني	*Dár-chee-nee* Cinnamon
رازيانه	*Ra-zeĕ-á neh* A species of aniseed
زراوند	*Zir-a-wund* Birthwort
زعفران	*Zá-frán* Saffron
زيرا	*Zee-ra* Cumin seed

شاهترا	*Shah-tereh* Fumitory
صعتر	*Sââ-tur* Origany, or wild thyme
عود	*Oowd* Lignum aloes
غاريقون	*Ghá-ree-koon* Agaric
فراسيون	*Frá-see-yoon* Euphrasia, eye-bright
قردمانا	*Koor-du-má-ná* Cardmine
قنطوريون	*Kun-too-ree-yoon* Centaury
كبابه	*Ku-bá-beh* Cubebs
كرفس	*Kerefs* Parsley
كرسنه	*Kir-us-neh* Peas
كشوث	*Koo-shoofs* The herb curfuta
مرزنجوش	*Mir-zun-joosh* Marjoram
نانخواه	*Nán-kháh* A species of cumin seed
هليون	*Hul-yoon* Asparagus

ملطفات

ملطفات *MU-LUTTIFAT.*——ATTENUANTIA.

ابهل	*Ub-hel* Fruit of the plane tree		خردل	*Khir-dul* Muſtard ſeed
انخر	*Iz-keir* Camel's hay		دارچيني	*Dár-chee-nee* Cinnamon
اسطوخودوس	*Us-too-khoo-doos* Stoechas		زراوند	*Zir-á-wund* Birthwort
اثقيل	*Iſs-keel* Squills		زوفاءخشك	*Zoofá-khooſhk* Hyſſop·
اقحوان	*Ok-hy-wân* Lovage		سداب	*Sudâb* Rue
انجره	*Un-je-reh* Nettle		سركه	*Seer-keh* Vinegar
ايرسا	*Iyr-ſa* Root of blue Iris		سكبينج	*Sug-bee-nuj* Sagapenum
بابونه	*Bá-boo-neh* Camomile flowers		سير	*Seer* Garlic
بوره	*Boo-reh* Borax		صعتر	*Sââ-tur* Origany
پودنه	*Pow-de-neh* Mint		عاترقرحا	*Akir-kir-hâ* Pellitory
جعده	*Joá-deh* A ſpecies of wormſeed		فنجنكشت	*Funj-ungooſht* The chaſte tree
جندبيدستر	*Joond-bey-duſter* Civet		قردمانا	*Koor-du-mâ-nâ* Cardmine
حاشا	*Há-ſhá* Thyme		قرطم	{ *Koor-tim* Safflower, baſtard ſaffron
حب‌البان	*Hub-ul-bán* Ben nuts		مشكطارامشيع	*Miſhkē-toorâ-miſh-eeyâ* Dittany
حرف	*Hoorf* Seed of Garden creſſes		كمادريوس	*Ku-má-dree-yoos* Germander.
حرمل	*Hirmul* Wild rue			
حماض	*Hum-âz* Sorrel			

مدرات *MÚ-DORRÁT*——STIMULANTIA.

ابهل	*Ubhel* Fruit of the plane tree		برنجاسف	*Bir-un-jâ-ſif* Mugwort
اقحوان	*Ok-hywân* Lovage		بابونه	*Bâ-boo-neh* Camomile flowers
انجدان	{ *Un-je-dân* The ſeed of the aſafœtida plant		پرسياوشان	*Pir-ſy-ow-ſhân* Maiden hair
انيسون	*Á-nee ſoon* Aniſeed		تخم كزر	*Tokhem Guz-ir* Carrot ſeed

ترمس

ترمس	*Toor-mi's* Egyptian lupin
جاوشیر	*Já-wé-sheer* Gum opopanax
جعده	*Joá-deh* A species of wormseed
جندبیدستر	*Joond-bey-duster* Civet
حبةالخضرا	{ *Hubbet ûl khûz-rah* Fruit of the turpentine tree
نانخواه	{ *Nán-kháh* A species of cumin seed
دارچینی	*Dár-chee-nee* Cinnamon
رازیانه	{ *Rá-zee-áneh* A species of aniseed
زوفاءخشك	*Zoofa Khooshk* Hyssop
سداب	*Sudáb* Rue
سعد	*Saad* A prickly grass
سلیخه	*Sé-lee-kheh* Cassia lignum
شونیز	*Show-neez* A small black seed
عروق	*Ou-rook* Sulphur

بابونه	*Bá-booneh* Camomile flowers
عود	*Owd* Lignum aloes
فراسیون	{ *Frá-see-yoon* Euphrasia, eye-bright
قردمانا	*Koor-du-má-ná* Cardmine
قسط	*Cost* Costus
قنطوریون	*Kun-tooryoon* Centaury
کبابه	*Kub-á-beh* Cubebs
کرفس	*Kerefs* Parsley
کمادریوس	*Kum-á-dry-oos* Germander
مرزنجوش	*Mir-zun-joosh* Marjoram
مشكطارامشیع	*Mishké-toorá-my-sheé-á* Dittany
میعه	*Mee-áh* Storax
نمام	*Ne-mám* Mother of thyme.

MU-FUTTÉ-TÁT.——LITHONTRIPTICA. مفتتات

اسارون	*Á-sa-roon* Asarabacca
بادام تلخ	*Bá-dám telkh* Bitter almond
برنجاسف	*Bir-un-ja-sif* Mugwort
پرسیاوشان	*Pir-sy-ow-shán* Maiden hair
تخم خربزه خشك	{ *Tokhem Khurboozèh khooshk* Dried musk-melon seed

حجرالیهود	*Hejr-ul-yehood* Jew's stone
رازیانه	{ *Rá zee-á-neh* A species of aniseed
سعد	*Saád* A prickly grass
سكبینج	*Sug-bee-nuj* Sagapenum
صمغ آلو	*Sum-egh áloo* Plum-tree gum
نخودسیاه	*Nákhood sy-ah* A species of vetch

قابضات

قابضات *KÁ-BIZ-ÁT.*——ASTRINGENTIA.

انخر	*Iz-kheir* Camel's hay	سماق	*Su-mâk* Sumach
امرود	*Umrood* Pear	طباشير	*Te-bâ-fheer* Sugar of bamboe
باقلا	*Bâ-ke-lâ* Beans	طين مختوم	*Teen Mukhtoom* Sealed earth
بيخ بارتنك	*Beykh Bûr-tung* Root of ribwort	عدس	*Ud-us* A fpecies of vetch
برنج	*Bě-runj* Rice	كرويا	*Kur-wee-ya* Caraway feed
ورق زر	*Werek zir* Gold leaf	كندر	*Koondir* Frankincenfe
بلوط	*Beloot* Acorns	كهربا	*Keh-robâ* Amber
بسد	*Boo-fud* Coral	كاورس	*Gâ-wirs* A fpecies of vetch
تخم شاهسفرم	{ *Tokhem fhâhus-fe-rum* Seed of fweet bafil	مصطكي	*Moos-tè-kà* Gum maftich
تخم كل	*Tokhem gool* Rofe feed	مورد	*Mow-rud* Myrtle
جوزسرو	{ *Fawz fir-oe* Fruit of the cyprefs tree	ناردين	*Nârdeen* Celtic nard
دم الاخوين	*Dum ul akhwein* Dragon's blood	نشاسته	*Nĕ-fhâs-teh* Starch
زعرور	*Za-roor* Medlars	نبق	*Nibk* A fpecies of lote
		نخود	*Nekhood* A fpecies of vetch

محللات *MO-HELIL-ÁT.*——DISCUTIENTIA.

انخر	*Iz-kheir* Camel's hay	بابونه	*Bâ-boo-neh* Camomile flowers
اسقيل	*Is-keel* Squills	برنجاسف	*Bir-un-ja-fif* Mugwort
إسارون	*A-sâ-roon* Afarabacca	پرسياوشان	*Pir-fy-ow-fhân* Maiden hair
انشق	*Oufhuc* Gum ammoniacum	پودنه	*Powdeneh* Mint
اقحوان	*Ok-hywân* Lovage	ترمس	*Toor-mifs* Egyptian lupin
اكليل الملك	*Ukleel ul mě-lic* Melilot	جعده	*Joe-deh* A fpecies of wormfeed
باقلا	*Bâ-ke-lâ* A fpecies of bean	جاوشير	*Jâ-we-fheer* Gum opopanax

F   حاشا

حاشا	*Há-shá* Thyme	عار	*Ghár* Laurel
خرزهره	*Khir-zereh* Rhododaphne	قثا	*Kissa* The long cucumber
خروع	*Khir wá* Palma christi	قنه	*Koon-neh* Galbanum
خطمي	*Khit-mee* A species of Mallows	كبر	*Kub-ir* Capers
روباه ترببك	*Robah-tirbuc* A species of nightshade	كمات	*Ké-mát* A species of fungus
زراوند	*Zir-á-wund* Birthwort	لادن	*Lá-dun* The herb labdanum
زفت	*Zift* Pitch	كمادريوس	*Kemá-dryoos* Germander
سوسن	*So-sun* Lily	مرزنجوش	*Mir-zun-joosh* Marjoram
صمغ بطم	*Sumegh bootem* Gum of the turpentine tree	نمام	*Némám* Mother of thyme

منضجات *MUN-ZIJ-ÁT*——SUPPURANTIA.

اكليل الملك	*Ukleel ul melic* Melilot	كرنب	*Kir-nub* Cabbage
انجير	*Unjeer* Figs	لادن	*Lá-dun* Labdanum
ايرسا	*Iyr-sa* Root of blue Iris	مر	*Murr* Myrrh
برك خطمي	*Birg Khitmee* Mallow leaves	مرورشك	*Mirwir-shuck* An odoriferous grass
زعفران	*Zá-frán* Saffron	موم	*Moom* Bees' wax
صمغ بطم	*Sumegh bootem* Gum of the turpentine tree	ميعه	*Mee-áh* Storax

مغشيات *MO-FE-SHY-AT*——CARMINATIVA.

افتيمون	*Afteemoon* Dodder of thyme	پنجنكشت	*Punj-ungoosht* Agnus castus
انيسون	*A-nce-soon* Aniseed	تخم گزر	*Tokhem guz-zir* Carrot seed
بسباسه	*Biss-bá-seh* Mace	جاوشير	*Já-we-sheer* Opopanax

حماما

حماما *Hē-má-má* Amomum	سعد *Saad* Roots of a species of grass
دارفلفل *Dár filfil* Long pepper	صعتر *Sá-tur* Origany
زراوند *Zir-á-wund* Birthwort	فلفل *Filfil* Black pepper
زرنباد *Zir-em-bád* Zedoary	قردمانا *Koor-du-má-ná* Cardmine
زنجبيل *Zunjebeel* Dried ginger	كرفس *Kerefs* Parsley
زيره *Zee-rah* Cumin seed	نانخواه {*Nán-kháh* A species of Wormseed
سداب *Sudáb* Rue	

مقويات دماغ *MO-KE-WY-ÁT DEMÁGH*——CEPHALICA.

آملج *Ám-luj* Emblic Myrobolans	عود *Owd* Lignum aloes
انفخه ضان {*Unfekheh zán* Rennet of an ewe	عنبر *Umbir* Ambergris
بالنكو {*Bá-lun-goo* A species of sweet basil	غاليه {*Gha-leah* A composition of musk, ambergris, camphor, and oil of ben nuts
بلادر {*Eé-lá-door* Anacardium, Malacca bean	قرنفل *Kir-un-ful* Cloves
بندق *Bin-dook* Filberts	كندر *Koondir* Frankincense
بهاربه وامرود وسيب {*Báhar beeh wu umrood wu seeb* Blossoms of quinces, pears, and apples	كل سرخ *Gool Soorkh* Red roses
دماغ حيوانات {*Demágh hywán-át* The brains of animals	لبن ضان *Lebn zán* Ewe's milk
روغن عنبر *Roghen umbir* Oil of ambergris	لحم دراج *Lehm dir-ráj* The flesh of quail
زنجبيل *Zun-je-beel* Dried ginger	لحم دجاج {*Lehm Dujaj* Flesh of the house hen
سعد *Saad* Roots of a species of grass	ماء الورد *Má-ul-wird* Rose Water
سيب *Seeb* Apples	مشك *Mooshk* Musk
سنبل *Sembul* Spikenard	نسرين *Nusreén* The wild rose
شربت نارنج *Shirbut nárenj* Orange sherbet	ياسمين *Ye-ás-meen* Jasmine

ابريشم

مقوبات‌دل MO-KÉ-WY-ÁT DIL.——CARDIACA.

ابریشم	*Ub-rey-fhem* Raw filk		سوسن	*So-fun* Lily
اترج	*Ut-rej* Citron		سیب	*Seeb* Apples
اسطوخودوس	*Is-too-khoodoos* Stoechas		شغاقل	*She-ká-kul* Wild carrot
امرود	*Umrood* Pears		صندل	*Sundel* Sandal wood
امله	*Ám-leh* Emblic myrobalans		طباشیر	*Te-bá-fheer* Sugar of bamboo
انار شیرین	*Ánár fhereen* Sweet pome-granates		طین مختوم	*Teen Mukhtoom* Sealed earth
بادروج	*Bádrooj* A fpecies of fweet bafil		عنبر	*Umbir* Ambergris
بالنگو	*Bá-lun-goo* An odoriferous plant		عود	*Ood* Lignum aloes
بسفایج	*Bis-fa-yej* Polypody		فرنجمشك	*Ferenjmoofhk* An odoriferous plant
بسد	*Boos-fud* Coral		قاقله	*Ká-ke-leh* Cardamums
به	*Beeh* Quince		كافور	*Ká-foor* Camphor
پوست‌اترج	*Poaft Utrij* Citron peel		كشنیزخشك	*Kifhneez khoofhk* Dried cori-ander feed
تمرهندی	*Temr-hindee* Tamarind		كهربا	*Keh-ro-bá* Amber
جدوار	*Jedwár* A fpecies of ginger		كاوزبان	*Gow-ze-bán* Buglofs, ox tongue
دارچینی	*Dár-chee-nee* Cinnamon		كلسرخ	*Gool foorkh* Red rofe
درونج	*Diroo-nuj* A root refembling the tail of a fcorpion		لاجورد	*Láj-wird* Lapis lazuli
ریباس	*Ree-báfs* Rhapontic		لولو	*Loo-loo* Pearl
زرنباد	*Zir-um-bad* Zedoary		مورد	*Mow-rud* Myrtle
زعفران	*Zá-frán* Saffron		نمام	*Ne-mám* Mother of thyme
سعد	*Saad* Roots of a fpecies of grafs		نارمشك	*Nár-moofhk* A fragrant flow-er, commonly called *ná-gifsir*
سلیخه	*Sé-lee-kheh* Caffia lignea		نعناع	*Ná-naá* Spearmint
سنبل	*Sembul* Spikenard			

نیلوفر

نيلوفر	*Nee-loo-fir* Water lily	هليله	*He-lee-leh* Yellow myrobalans
ورق زرونقره	{ *Werek zir wu nokerah* Gold and silver leaf	ياقوت	*Yá-coot* Ruby

---

مقويات كبد   *MO-KÉ-WY-AT* KÉBID.——HEPATICA.

اشنه	*Oushneh* Dodder of oak, &c.		smell, and is therefore also called *Kirfetúl ke-run-full*, or *bark of cloves*: another spe-
اظفاالطيب	*Uzfár ul teib* Perfumed nails		cies is thinner, of a brighter
جوزبوا	*Jowz bu-wá* Nutmeg		red, and sweeter to the taste,
حب البلسان	*Hubul Bulesán* Carpobalsam		resembling small pieces of
حماما	*Humámá* Amomum		cinnamon, but the first kind
دارچيني	*Dárcheenee* Cinnamon		is preferable.
غافث	*Ghá-fis* Hemp agrimony	كشوث	*Ku-shoos* A species of Dodder
قرنفل	*Ke-run-full* Cloves	مصطكي	*Mustē-ká* Mastich
قرفه	*Kirfeh* An odoriferous thick bark, of the colour of cloves, which it also resembles in	ناردين	*Nárdain* Celtic nard

---

مقويات معده   *MO-KÉ-WY-ÁT* ME-OA-DEH.——TONICA.

امله	*Ám-leh* Emblic myrobalans	سعد	*Sáad* Roots of a species of grass
انخر	*Iz-kier* Camel's hay	سفرجل	*Suf-er-jel* Quince
بالنكو	*Bálungoo* A species of sweet basil	سلينخه	*Se-lee-kheh* Cassia lignea
بليله	*Be-le-leh* Belleric myrobalans	سباق	*Sumák* Sumach
پوست ترنج	*Poast Turenj* Citron peel	طباشير	*Te-bá-sheer* Sugar of bamboe
جوزبوا	*Jowz-bu-wá* Nutmeg	قاقله	*Ká-ku-leh* Cardamoms
دارچيني	*Dárcheenee* Cinnamon	قرنفل	*Ke-run-full* Cloves
زرنباد	*Zer-em-bád* Zedoary	قرفه	{ *Kirfeh* An odoriferous bark, *vide supra*
سادج هندي	*Sádij hindee* Indian leaf	كل سرخ	*Goolsoorkh* Red rose

G

كرويا

كرويا	*Kur-wee-yá* Caraways	مصطكي	*Mus-tĕ-ká* Maſtich
كندر	*Keondir* Frankincenſe	نعناع	*Na-ráá* Mother of thyme
مشكطارامشيع	*Miſk-ketrá-meſhyá* Dittany	هليله	*He-lee-leh* Yellow myrobalans

مبهيات MO-BÉHY-ÁT.——APHRODISIACA.

انجير	*Injeer* Figs	شقاقل	*Shĕ-ká-kul* Wild carrot
رطب	*Ru-teb* Freſh dates	شيرميش	*Sheer meeſh* Ewe's milk
بسباسه	*Bir-báfsá* Mace	فستق	*Fis-took* Piſtachio nuts
انكور	*Ungoor* Grapes	فندق	*Findook* Filberts
باقلا	*Eá-kĕ-lá* A ſpecies of bean	قرفه	{ *Kir feh* An odoriferous bark, *vide Hepatica*
بيضه كبوتر	*Byzĕh ke-boo-tir* Pigeon's eggs	قسط	*Kuſi* Coſtus
بيضه كبك	*Byzĕh Kulk* Partridge's eggs	كثيرا	*Ke-fee-rá* Gum tragacanth
بيضه كنجشك	*Byzĕh kunjeſhk* Sparrow's eggs	اكر	*Ig-gir* Sweet-ſcented flag
پنيرمايه شتر	{ *Pun-cer-máyeh ſhootir* Rennet of a camel	كرفس	*Kerefs* Parſley
جرجير	*Jir-jeer* A kind of bean	كنجد	*Kun-jid* Sefamé
چلغوزه	{ *Chulgkoozeh* Fruit of the mountain pine	كزر	*Guz-ir* Carrot
حبةالخضرا	{ *Hubbetál khuzrá* Fruit of the turpentine tree	لوبيا	*Loo by á* A ſpecies of bean
حلتيت	*Hilteet* Aſafœtida	مغزجوز	*Meghz jowz* Peeled walnuts
خصيةالثعلب	*Khuſiyet 'l' ſáieb* Satyrion	مغزبادام	{ *Meghz Bá-dám* Bleeched almonds
خولنجان	*Khoolinján* Galangal	مغزدماغ كنجشك وبره	{ *Meghz demagh khunjiſhk wu bu-reh* Brains of ſparrows, and of kid
دارچيني	*Dárcheenee* Cinnamon	نارجيل	*Nâr-jeel* Cocoa nut
زرنباد	*Zer en bád* Zedoary	هليون	*Hulyoon* Aſparagus
زنجبيل	*Zunjebeel* Dried ginger	نخود	*Nákhood* A ſpecies of vetch
سقنقور	*Suck-un-koor* Skink		
سورنجان	*Soor-in-ján* Hermodactyls		

مسكنات اوجاع

مسكنات اوجاع *MO-SUCKEN-ÁT OWJÁ.*——ANODYNA.

اسغيداج	*Is-fy.dáj* White lead	
افيون	*Ufi-oon* Opium	
بيخ بيروج	{ *Beykh Beyrooj* Root of the mandrake	
پيهبط	*Peeh but* Goofe greafe	
تورک	*Tooruck* Purflain	

سغيده تخم مرغ	{ *Sefeydeh tokhem murgh* White of egg
صمغ عربي	*Semegh árebee* Gum Arabic
كثبرا	*Ke-fee-ra* Gum tragacanth
نشاسته	*Nefhájteh* Starch

مسبتنات *MO-SE-BÉ-TÁT.*——HYPNOTICA.

اصطرک	*Us-te-ruck* Storax	
اقحوان	*Owk-hy-wán* Lovage	
حاما	*Hʊmá-má* Amomum	
زعفران	*Záf-rán* Saffron	
شاهسفرم	*Sháhusferem* Sweet bafil	
شبت	*Shib-it* Fennel	

شقايق	*She-ká-yik* Anemone
حلتيت	*Hilteet* Afafœtida
كاهو	*Kù-hu* Lettuce
لغاح	*Lu-fah* Fruit of the mandrake
مرو	*Merow* A berry

قاطعات ديدان *KÁ-TÉ-ÁAT DEE-DAN.*——ANTHELMINTICA.

اثمد	*Is-mud* Native antimony	
افسنتين	*Afsunteen* Wormwood	
برنج كابلي	*Beerʊnj Cábulee* A black feed refembling pepper, only	

smaller; it is white within-fide, and a little bitter

جعده	*Joa-deh* A fpecies of wormfeed
زوفاي خشك	*Zoofa khoofhk* Hyffop.

مانعات رعاف واسهال الدم *MÁ-NYÁT RO-ÁF WU ISS-HÁL-UD'-DUM.* STYPTICA.

اثمد	*Is-mud* Native antimony	
بادروج	*Bád-rooj* A fpecies of fweet bafil	

بزر البنيج	*Buz-ir ul Eʊnj* Henbane feed
بلوط	*Beloot* Acorns

تينم كرل

تنخم كل	*Tokhem gool* Rose seed	كشنيز	*Kishneez* Coriander seed
جوزسرو	{ *Jowz sir-oe* Fruit of the cypress tree	كهربا	*Keh-ro-bá* Amber
حضض	*Hu-zuz* Juice of buck thorn	كلنار	{ *Goolnár* Flowers of the fruitless pomegranate
دم الاخوين	*Dum-ul-áhkwain* Dragon's blood	كل ارمني	*Gil urmenee* Bole armenic
ريوند	{ *Rey-wend* Rhapontic, wild rhubarb	لسان الحمل	{ *Lissán ul heml* Ribwort, or plantain
زرشك	*Zir-ushk* Barberries	مازو	*Má-zou* Gall apple
زيره	*Zeerah* Cumin seed	مصطكي	*Mustē-ká* Mastich
شادنه	*Shá-dē-neh* Bloodstone	نشاسته	*Neshásteh* Starch
قنطوريون	*Kun-teeryoon* Centaury	نعناع	*Na-náâ* Mother of thyme
كافور	*Ká-foor* Camphor		

مقرحات MO-KÉ-RE-HÁT.——VESCEATORIA

اسقيل	*Is-keil* Squills	سداب	*Sud-áb* Rue
اهك	*Áhúck* Quick lime	سنباده	*Sum-bá-deh* Emery stone
بورق	*Booruc* Borax	صابون	*Sá-boon* Soap
حرف	*Hoorf* Seed of garden cresses	فربيون	*Fir-byoon* Euphorbium
ذراريح	*Ze-rá-reeh* Cantharides	قسط	*Kust* Costus
راسن	*Rá-sun* Elecampane	تلقطارسبز	*Kul-kē-trá subz* Green vitriol
زاج	*Zaj* White vitriol	لبن يتوع	{ *Lebn ye-tua* Milky juice of plants
زرنيخ	*Zir-neikh* Arsenic		

مدملات قروح MO-DUM-IL-ÁT KE-ROUH.——CICATRIZANTIA.

اثمد	*Is-mud* Native antimony	ايرسا	*Iyr-sa* Iris root
اسرنج	*Iss-renj* Red lead	دم الاخوين	*Dumulákhwain* Dragon's blood
		انزروت	

انزروت	*Unzeroot* Sorcocolla	طبين مختوم	*Teen mukhtoom* Sealed earth
زراوند	*Zir-á-wend* Birthwort	عسل	*Afful* Honey
زيره	*Zeerah* Cumin feed	كلنار	*Goolnár* Pomegranate bloſſoms
صبر	*Syb-ir* Aloes	لسان الحمل	*Liſſun ul hēml* Ribwort
صمغ آلو	*Semegh aloo* Plum-tree gum	ورق بلوط	*Werek beloot* Oak leaves

مجليات اوساخ قروح *MOƷELLYÁT OIWSÁK KEROUH.*—DETERGENTIA.

ايهل	*Ubhel*	حب بلسان	*Hub buleſán* Carpobalſam
آبكامه	*Ab-ká-meh* A compoſition of milk curds, and feed of wild rue, prepared with leaven and vinegar	راتينج	*Rá-te-nej* Reſin
		زفت	*Ziſt* Pitch
		عسل	*Aſſul* Honey
ايرسا	*Iyr-ſa* Iris root	نمك	*Né-muck* Salt

اكال كوشت زياده قروح *ÁKÁL COWSHT ZÝADEH KEROUH.*-CAUSTICA.

انزروت	*Unzeroot* Sorcocolla	صوف سوخنه	*Soof ſowkhteh* Burnt wool
توبال مس	*Tobál miſs* Blue vitriol	مرد ارسنك	*Moordár ſung* Litharge of lead
زنكار	*Zun-gár* Verdegris		

يابسات قروح *YÁ-BIS-ÁT KEROUH.*——EPULOTICA.

اشنه	{ *Ouſhneh* Moſs of pine, and other trees	اهك شسة	*Áhuck ſhoos-teh* Slacked lime
		توتيا	*Too-ty-á* Tutty
خرماي سوخته	*Khoorma ſokhteh* Burnt dates	صبر	*Syb-ir* Aloes
انزروت	*Unzeroot* Sorcocolla	صوف سوخته	*Soof Sokhteh* Burnt wool

H

پوست انار

پوست انار	*Poost anár* Pomegranate peel	سرکه ونوشادر و نمك	*Seer-keh wu nowshádir, wu ne-muck* A mixture of vinegar, fal ammoniac, and falt
زاك سوخته	*Zág fewkhteh* Burnt alum	سورنجان	*Soor in-ján* Hermodactyls
زنکار با سپده بیضه مرغ سرشته	*Zun-gár bá fepeydeh Byzeh murgh ferifhteh* Verdegris with white of egg	صعتر	*Sá-tur* Origany

ادویه هیضه *ADVIYAH HEE-ZEH.*——STOMACHICA.

ابی وسیب بریان کرده	*Ab-ee wu feeb be-ryán kirdeh* Fried quinces and apples	اقراص الطبین	*Ákráfs'ul teen* Lozenges made of boles
اب ابی ترش	*Áb áb-ee toorfh* Juice of four quinces	سویق	*Se-weyk* Fried barley
اب سیب کوهی	*Áb feeb kouhee* Juice of crab apple	حب الرمان	*Hub'ul rum-mán* Pomegranate feeds
اقراص مورد	*Ákráfs moorud* Myrtle lozenges	شراب میوها	*Sheráb meywá-há* All kinds of fruit wines
اقراص کندر	*Ákráfs koondir* Frankincenfe lozenges	صندل وکلاب	*Sundul wu gooláb* Sandal wood and rofe water
اقراص راسن	*Ákráfs rá fun* Elecampane lozenges	مورد وکلاب	*Moorud wú gooláb* Myrtle and rofe water

WEIGHTS.

WEIGHTS.

حبه *Hubbeh, a.* equal to one وجو *jow*, or common barley-corn.

تسو *Tuffoo, a.* — — 2 barley-corns.

قيراط *Keerat, a.* or *carat,* — 4 barley-corns.

كهونكهچي *Ghunghchy, h.* ⎫
سرخ *Soorkh, h.* -   ⎬ — 8 barley-corns.
رتي *Rutty, h.* -   ⎭

ماشه *Máfhah, h.* — — 8 rutties.

توله *Tolah, h.* — — 12 mafhahs.

تانك *Tánk, h.* — — 4 mafhahs.

دانك *Dáng, p.* ⎫
or   ⎬ — — 4⅙ rutties.
دانق *Dánek, a.* ⎭

درم *Direm, p.* ⎫
or   ⎬ — 1 mafhah and 1 rutty.
درهم *Dirhem, a.* ⎭

مثقال *Mifkál, a.* — 4 mafhahs and 3½ rutties.

استار *Iftár, a.* ⎫
or   ⎬ 1½ tolahs and 2 mafhahs.
سير شاهي *Seer Sháhy, h.* or, *royal feer.* ⎭

اوقيه *Owkyáh, a* ⎫
or   ⎬ — 7½ mifkals.
وقيه *Wekyáh, a.* ⎭

من طبي *Mun tibby, a.* 40 iftars.

ULFÁZ UDWIYEH

THE

MATERIA MEDICA.

ABBREVIATIONS.

a. Arabic. *g.* Greek. *ſy.* Syriac. *p.* Perſian. *h.* Hindevy. *v.* ordinary name. *qu.* quality.

1, 2, 3, 4, degrees. *prop.* medical properties. *ch.* what part or kind to be choſen. *cor.* correctors·

d. doſe. *ſuc.* ſuccedaneum.

---

(1) آارغيس AARGHEES. *g.* Bark of the root of the barberry buſh.

پوست بیخ درخت زرشک

p. poſt beykh diruckt ze-ruſhk.

(2) آطريلال A-TEREE-LÁL. Crowfoot.

تخم خلال خلبل رجل الغراب

a. rejel ul gherab.   *p. tokhem khelál kheleél.* काकजंत्री मीसी

h. kákjungee, and alſo *miſſee.*

qu. hot and dry 2. *ch.* the ſeed.

(3) آلسن Á-LE-SUN. Wild rue.

p. ſepund ſowkhtenee. سپند سوختني

(4) ابوخلسا ABOO KHULSÁ. A ſpecies of bugloſs.

شنکار *p. ſhunkár.*

qu. hot and dry 2. *ch.* black, with many leaves, and thick root. *d.* as far as 2 direms.

(5) ابرکاکیا ABERKÁKYÁ. *a.* Cobweb.

मकनेकाजाला تنيده عنکبوت

p. teneedeh unkáboot. *h. muckree ká jála.*

prop. uſed to ſtop bleeding at the noſe; and applied to green wounds that are ſuperficial.

(6) ابن الماء IBN-UL-MÁ. *a.* Any water fowl.

p. mor-

I

p. *murghábee.* مرغابي

The flesh is heating.

(7) آبست A-BIST. *a.* Pulp of citron. कॊ गो नेकागोद كوشت ترنج

p. *gowsht turenj.* h. *bee-jowré-ká good.*

   qu. hot and moist 1. *ch.* the species called *bálung.* vide 140.

(8) آبار A-BAR. *a.* Burnt lead. ददं سرب سوختنه

h. *bung.*   p. *soorbsowkhteh.*

   qu. cold and dry 2. *suc.* native antimony.

(9) ابغر UB-KIR. *a.* Nitre. लोजी h. *bá-jee.*   p. *shooreh* شوره

(10) ابرار UB-RAR. *a.* Houseleek. p. *hy-ul-aalum.* حي العالم

(11) ابن طاهر IBN TAHIR. *a.* Partridge.

p. *kubk.* كبك

(12) آبنوس ÁBNOOS. *a.* Ebony.

p. *aw-noos.* آونوس

   qu. hot and dry 2. *prop.* astringent and pungent. *ch.* black, and that will sink in water. *cor.* gum Arabic with sweet basil. *suc.* konar wood; or burnt date seed.

(13) ابو علس ABOO ULS. *a.* Name of a flower.

p. *gool khyree.* گل خيري

   qu. hot and dry 1. *prop.* drawing. *ch.* fresh gathered. *d.* a very small quantity. *cor.* yolk of egg.

(14) ابن عرس IBN URS. *a.* The mungoose.

निवॊउल h. *neywul.*   p. *rasoo.* راسو

   qu. flesh hot and dry. *prop.* attenuant. *ch.* that which is well covered with hair. *d.* one direm to one miskál, mixed with salt, may be taken to prevent the effects of pestilential air. *cor.* oils. *suc.* rennet, in cases of the epilepsy.

(15) آبق ÁBUC. *a.* Mercury.

पारा h. *pá-ra.*   p. *seem-áb.* سيماب

(16) ابهرک UBH-RUCK. Talc.

p. *tulc.* طلق

(17) ابهل UBHEL. *a.* The seed of the plane tree, and of the mountain pine.

तॊबीर तखमॊवहल-तखम सरॊकॊरुही تخم وهل - تخم سرو کوهي

p. *tokhem wowhel* and *tokhem sir-œ-kouhee.* h. *howh-beer.*

   qu. hot and dry 3 *prop.* diaphoretic and attenuant, and good for cleaning ulcers. *ch.* black and large, gathered from a tree with leaves of a golden colour. *d.* from two direms to a miskál. *cor.* lignum aloes, or galangal, or amomum, or barberries. *suc.* cypress kernels; or an equal weight of cassia lignea; or one and half direms of cinnamon.

(18) ابل EBIL. The lesser cardamom.

p. *ká-ke-leh seghár.* قاقله صغار

(19) ابابيل A-BA-BEEL. *a* The swallow.

सपाबीनी پرستوک

h. *s-pa-*

h. *ſe-pá-bee-nee.*   p. *pur-uſ-took.*

(20) ابریسم EB-REY-SUM. Raw ſilk.

पाठ h. *pautﬁ.*   p. *ebreyſhum.* ابریشم

(21) ابرون ABROON. Houſe leek.

p. *hy-ul-áálum.* حي العالم

(22) آبكون ABGOON   Starch.

गिहूंकाहीर h. *geehoon-ká-heer.*   p. *neſháﬂeh.* نشاستنه

(23) ابرارالقطه ABRAR ULKUT-EH.
Seed of houſe leek.

p. *tokhem hy ul áálum.* تخم حي العالم

(24) ابرهيميه IB-RE-HY-MEYAH.
A kind of broth.

(25) آبكامه AB-KA-MEH.   Bread
ſoaked in water, and kept in the ſun
till it becomes ſour.

h. *kán-jee.* कांजी

(26) آبكينه AB-GEE-NEH.   Glaſs.

कांच h. *kántch.*   p. *ſheeſheh.* شيشه

(27) ابن‌حبه IBN HUBBEH. *a.* Bread.

रोटी h. *roo-tee.*   p. *nan.* نان

(28) ابي A-BEE.   Quince

बिही
p. h. *be-hee.*   سفرجل   *a. ſuf-ir-jel.*

(29) ابن‌آوي IBN A-WEE.   The
jackal.

सीयाल — गीदर   شغال

h. *ſee-dl* and *gee-dir.*   p. *ſheghál.*

(30) اترج UT-REJ.   Citron.

बिजोरा h. *beyjowrá.*   p. *turenj.* ترنج

qu the peel is hot and dry 2; the inner white
coat, hot and moiſt 1; the juice, cold and dry 2;
the ſeed, hot and moiſt. *prop.* cardiac, tonic, attenuant, and diaphoretic. *ch.* large, with yellow
ſkin. *d.* for the bite of a ſcorpion, two miſkáls
of the ſeed may be taken infuſed in hot water.

31) اترار UT-RÁR.   Barberries.
p. *zer-uſhk.* زرشك

qu. cold and dry. *ch.* thoſe that are tranſparent.

(32) اتنامیس ÁT-NÁ-MEES. Wild
camomile.

p. *bábooneh burree.* بابونه‌بري

(33) اتان UT-ÁN.   A ſhe aſs.

गदहि   ماده‌خر

h. *gud-e-hee.*   p. *má-deh khur.*

(34) اثمد IS-MUD.   *a.* Native antimony.

इंजन   سنگ‌سرمه

h. *unjen.*   p. *ſung ſirmeh.*

qu. cold 1, dry 2.   *prop.* drying and ſtyptic.
ch. bright and brittle.   *cor.* ſugar, and coriander
ſeed.   *ſuc.* burnt lead.

(35) اثلق US-LUC.   *a.* Seed of agnus
caſtus.

संजालौके बिज

सनालो केबीज   تخم پنجنكشت
h. *fem-bha-loo ké beej.* p. *tokhem punj-ungoofht.*

(36) اثل US-EL. The tamarifk bufh.

ज्ञाबो h. *j-ha-ou.*   p. *guz.* کز

(37) اجلکیا AJEL GEE-A. *a.* A poi-fonous root.

बिस h. *bifs.*   p *beefh.* بیش

(38) اجبود UJ-MOOD. ब्रजमोद

A fpecies cf parfley.

p. *buz-ir-ul kerefs.*   بزرالكرفس

(39) اجاص E-JÁSS. A fpecies of plum.

आरो h. *ároo.*   p. *a-loo.* آلو

prop. emollient, and a good purgative of the bile.

(40) آجر A-JUR. Burnt bricks.

लकोरीईट   خشت پخته
h. *luck-howrec-eent.* p. *khifht pokhteh.*

prop. drying. *ch.* thofe that are new. *d.* one mifkál of the oil of bricks. *cor.* oil of violets. *f.* tiles.

(41) اجواین UJ-WA-IN. ब्रजवायन

A fpecies of anifeed.

p. *nan-khak.*   نانخواه

In Hindevy it moreover is called *jó-wá-én.*

(42) اجواین خراسانی *h.* UJ-WA-IN ब्रजवायनखरसानी
KHORASANY. Henbanefeed.

بزرالبنج   p. *buz-ir-ul bunj.*

(43) احلب دیای رومي EH-LUBDYA ROOMEE. A fpecies of fpurge.

v. *fhib-rim.*   شبرم

(44) احریض EH-REEZ. Safflower.

कोसंब: كاجیره
h. *kofumbh*   v. *kájee-reh.*

(45) احداق المرضي EH-DAK 'L'- MIRZA. Camomile flowers.

p. *babooneh gáw.*   بابونه کاو

(46) اخروت AKH-ROWT. ब्रखरोट Walnut.

جوز   چارمغز   کردکان
a. jowz. p. *char mughz.* and *geer di-gán.*

(47) اخکر ÁK-GIR. A live coal.

ब्रगारा   انكشت افروخته
h. *an-gá-rá*   p. *unkifht áfrokhteh*

(48) اخینوس EKHEENOOS. Wild wheat.

(49) اخریط EKHREET. Wild leek.

बंकागंदना   كندناي بري
h. *bun-ká gunde-ná.*   p. *gun-dé-ná bur-ree.*

(50) اخیل UKH-YUL. Name of a bird, whom the Arabians confider to be unlucky.

(51) اخزم UKH-ZUM. A young fnake.

p. *már*

p. *mar now.* مارنو

(52) اخیون UKH-YOON. *a.* Snake's head; name of a plant.

p. *ráss ul úf-e-iy.* راس الافعي

(53) اخبروسه UKH BÉ-RU-SEH. Wild wheat.

बनगेही दوسر کندم دشتي

h. *bun-gee-hoon.* v. p. *du-sir.* p. *gundum deshtee.*

(54) اداادا A-DÁ-DÁ. A species of mezereon.

p. *derukht kerem dáneh.* درخت کرم دانه

(55) آدا ÁDÁ. Green ginger.

श्रदरक श्रादा زنجبیل تر

h. *ád-ruck.* p. *zinjebeel tur.*

(56) ادرک ID-RICK. *a.* A small plum.

p. *áloo-cheh.* الوچه

(57) ادیچاره U-DE-CHÁ-REH. The inverted thorn.

चिचिरा خاروازکون

v. h. *chee-ché-ra.* p. *khár wagzoon.*

(58) ادراقي Á-DÁ-RÁ-KEE. *sy.* Name of a bitter root, very hard when dry.

कुचला فلوس ماهي

h. *kootchelá.* p. *fe-loos mdhee.*

(59) آذان الارنب AZÁN UL-ER-NUB. *a.* Hares' ears. A species of ribwort.

p. *we-rek bár-tung.* ورق بارتنک

(60) آذان الدب AZÁN ÚL DUB. *a.* Mullein. *p. goosh khyrs,* or bear's ears. کوش خرس

(61) آذان العبد AZÁN UL UBD. A species of shepherd's staff.

(62) آذان الغار AZÁN UL FAR. *a.* Mouse ear. p. *merjan goosh.*

مرزانکوش

qu. hot and dry 2. *d.* half a direm.

(63) اذخر IZ-KEER. *a.* Camel's hay.

रोधबिल کورکیا & کاهمکي

h. *gund beyl.* p. *gowr-gee-á,* and *ká-muck-ee.*

(64) آذریاس ÁZREE-YASS. Gum of wild rue. صمغ سداب کوهي

p. *semegh sudáb kou-hee.*

(65) آذان القیس AZÁN UL KÉ-SEES. *a.* A species of house-leek.

(66) اذناب الخیل UZNÁB UL KYEL. *a.* The plant horse tail.

सिरेसकागाच

h. *see-rs ká gátch.* p. *ás-lunj.*

K (67)

(67) آذان الغيل AZÁN UL FEEL. *a.*
Drangwort.

p. *pulgoosh,* and *loof.* لوف — پیلکوش

(68) آذان الغزال AZÁN UL GHÉ-
ZÁL. *a.* A species of buglofs.

(69) آذارافيون AZÁR-Á-FYOON.
A species of foam of the fea.

(70) آذريون AZREEYOON. Accor-
ding to fome, the anemone; others
fay it is the camomile plant.

(71) آذريو AZIR-YOU. The fun-
flower.

(72) آذان الجدي AZÁN UL JE-
DEE. *a.* Ribwort, arnogloffa.

p. *liffan ul heml.* لسان الحمل

(73) ارطاماسيا ÁRTE-MA-SY-Á. Ar-
temefia, mugwort.

p. *bir-un-ja-fif.* برنجاسف

(74) ارسطا ÁRIS-TÁ. Henbane.

p. *bung.* بنک

(75) ارسطلوخيا ARISTÁLOO-
KHEEÁ. Long birthwort.

p. *zerewend teweel.* زراوندطويل

(76) ارمينا URMEENÁ. Sal ammoniac. p. *nowfhadir.* نوشادر

(77) آراقوا ÁRA-KOO-WÁ. A weed
that grows amongſt wheat.

किका سهکک کندم

p. *fehuck gundum.* h. *keeká.*

(78) اروسا E-RU-SA. ब्रोसा & बोसा
An Indian plant, called alfo *bunfá.*

(79) ارقب ER-KUB. The mountain
goat. p. *búz kou-hee.* بزکوهي

(80) ارزت IR-ZUT. A fpecies of fir.
p. *fe-no-bér bey bir.* درختصنوبربيبر
The fir that does not bear fruit.

(81) اريدبريد Á-REED-BÁ-REED.
A root which refembles a fplit onion.
It is a native of *Seiftan.*

(82) ارشد UR-SHUD. The marcafite
ſtone.

v. *mir-ká-fhee-fhd.* مرقشيشا
qu. hot and dry 2.

(83) ارثد UR-SUD. The chafte tree.

संनालु پنجنکشت
p. *punjun goofht.* h. *fumbháloo.*

(84) ارند A-RUND. ब्रेंड palma
chrifti. p. *beed injeer.* بيدانجير

(85) ارز ÁRUZ. Rice.

चाबल h. *chá-wul.* p. *be-renj.* برنج
(86)

(86) ارزيز UR-ZEEZ. *p.* Tin.

रांगा رصاص قلعى

h. * rán-ga.* v. *ku-lie.* a. *re-sáss.*

(87) ارماط UR-MAT. Name of a flower.

कैवरेकाफूल h. *kew-reh ka'fhool.*

(88) ارقط UR-KUT. The leopard.

p. *pe-lung.* پلنك

(89) ارماك UR-MÁK. Name of a tree.

कैवरेकागाच h. *kew-reh ka gatch.*

(90) اراك UR-ÁK. *a.* A tree, of whose roots are made tooth-picks.

पिलुकागाच h. *pe-loo ka gatch.*

qu. hot and dry, 1.—*prop.* deobstruent.—*ch.* fragrant.—*d.* of the fruit 1 miskál.

(91) ارمال رومي UR-MÁL ROO-MEE. An aromatic bark of a tree growing in Yemen.

(92) اردم رومي UR-DUM-ROO-MEE. The anemone.

v. *ázree-yoon.* آنریون

(93) ارقم URKUM. A snake, black and white. p. *mar ubluck.* مارابلق

(94) ارمانيقون UR-MÁ-NEE-KOON. Henbane seed.

p. *buz-ir ul bunj.* بزرالبنج

(95) ارقان UR-KÁN. A species of privet.

मिन्दी h. *mhindee.* v. p. *hennah.* حنا

(96) اردشيران UR-DE-SHEERAN. A tree resembling jasmine.

(97) اربيان UR-BEE-YAN. A shrimp.

झिंगा ملخ دریایي

h. *jhinga.* p. *melekh de ry-a-i.*

(98) ارجان UR-JÁN. Wild almond.

जंगलीबादाम بادام كوهي

h. *jungelee ba-dam.* p. *ba-dám kou-hee.*

(99) ارجوان UR-JOO-WÁN. A tree bearing a beautiful purple flower.

p. *ur-ghé-wán.* ارغوان

qu. cold and dry.

(100) ارمنين UR-ME-NEEN. Wild pomegranate.

जंगलीअनार انارشتي قلقل

h. *jungelee anár.* a. *kilkul.* p. *anár deshtee.*

(101) ارسانيقون UR-SA-NEE-KOON. Yellow orpiment.

हरनाल زرنيخ زرد

h. *bir-tál.* p. *zir-neikh zird.*

(102)

(102) ارسغیلون UR-SE-KE-LOON. The same.

(103) ارزن AR-ZUN. A kind of millet. बिना h. chey-ná.

(104) اراہ Á-RÁH. Gum maftich.

(105) ارجیقنه UR-JEE-KE-NEH. A yellow grafs ufed in dying.

श्रसेपनक زریر h. as-pe-ruck. p. zé-reer.

(106) اردفناني IR-UD-FE-NÁ-NEE. v. Wild cucumber.

(107) ارنببری UR-NUB-BIR-REE. The hare. सता خرکوش h. fúffa'. p. khur-goofh.

(108) ارنببحري UR-NUB BEH-REE. The fea hare, a poifonous fifh, refembling a fhell.

(109) ارطي IR-TEE. The white poplar. v. fepeid-ár. سپیدار

(110) ارغاموني UR-GHÁ-MOO-NEE. A flower refembling the anemone.

(111) ازورد UZ-WIRD. The lote tree.

(112) اسموسا US-MOO-SÁ. Wild carrot.

(113) اسطرخا US-TIR-KHÁ. Red orpiment. मैन्सल زرنیخسرخ h. mynful. p. zir-neikh foorkh.

(114) اسپند ISS-PUND. Seed of wild rue. v. hir-mul. حرمل

(115) استهخرما US-TEH KHURMA. Date ftone.
prop. when burnt, it is drawing and detergent.

(116) اسرب US-RUB. A Lead.

(117) اسغیداج IS-FEE-DÁJ. White lead.

(118) اسغلنج IS-FE-LUNJ. The fhrub horfe tail, or goat's beard.

(119) اسغنج IS-FUNJ. Sponge. मुवाबादल ابرمرده h. moowa bá-dul. p. abir-moordeh.

(120) اسرنج IS-RINJ. Red lead. सेंदोर h. feindur.
prop. drying. ch. a bright red. fuc. white lead.

(121) اسغاناج IS-FÁ-NÁJ. Spinnage. साग पालक اسپاناج h. fág pá-luck. p. is-pá-náj.
prop. cool and emollient. cor. pepper. fuc. long cucumber; and purflain.

(122) اسودسالخ US-WUD SÁ-LIKH. A black fnake.

कालानाग

कालानाग ماريسياه

h. *kállá nág.* p. *már sy-ah.*

(123) اسغند سفيد IS-FUND-SE-FEID. A species of mustard-seed.

इसबंद تخم سپندان

h. *is-bund.* p. *tokhum se-pen-dan.*

prop. anodyne.

(124) اسد USSUD. The lion.

बाघ h. *bgáh.* p. *sheer.* شير

(125) استهول كند IS-THOOL-KUND. ब्रस्थोलकंद An Indian root.

(126) اسقنقور ISS-KUN-KOOR. The shink.

रेतमछली ريك ماهي نهنك دشتي

h. *reyt mutch-lee.* p. *reig máhee,* and *ne-heng desh-tee.* v. *se-kunkoor.* سقنقور

(127) اسمار IS-MÁR. Myrtle.

(128) اسطوخودوس US-TOO-KOO-DOOS. Stoechas.

(129) اسبيوس US-YOOS. Fixt alkaline salt. h. *cheen ka loon.* चीनकालोन

(130) اسغيوس ISS-FÉ-YOOS. Seed of fleawort.

(131) اسغاقس ISS-KA-KIS. A species of millet.

(132) اسقولوس US-KOO-LOOS. A plant, whose root is very viscous.

घासरस كياه سريشم

h. *gá-hss sir-eyss.* p. *gee-áh sir-ey-shum.*

(133) استطلس ISS-TUT-LUS. Jew's pitch.

(134) اسقوريدوس US-KOO-REE-DOOS. Rennet in general.

انفخه پنيرمايه

v. *un-fe-keh.* p. *pu-neer-máyeh.*

(135) اسطرماطوس US-TIR-MÁ-TOOS. Wild rue. اسبند

(136) اسد الارض USSUD UL URZ. The chameleon.

गरगिट حربا بوقلمون

h. *geer-git.* p. *boo-ke-le-moon.* v. *hir-bá.*

The chymists give this name also to quick-silver, on account of its assuming so many forms.

(137) استرنك US-TRUNG. Mandrake.

लछमनालछमनी یبروج p. مردم كيا

h. *luckmun-á luck-mu-nee.* v. *yeb-rooj.*

p. *mir-dum gee-á.*

(138) اسپرك AS-PE-RUCK. Melilot.

ब्रमपरक

(139) اسقبيل IS-KEEL. Squill.

कांदा *kándá.* *peyáz deshtee.* پياز دشتي

(140) اسفرم IS-FE-REM. Myrtle.

L

(141)

(۱٤۱) استقولوقندریون US-KOO-LOO-
KOON-DIR-YOON. Spleenwort.

(۱٤۲) اسارون Á-SÁ-ROON. Afara-
baca. तकर h. *tuckir.*

(۱٤۳) استقورون US-KOO-ROON.
Ruft of iron.

خبث الحدید a. *khubs'l' hé-deed.* ریم اهن p. *reem á-hun.*
किठ h. *keeth.*

(۱٤٤) اسطغنلین IS-TUF-LEEN.
Carrot.

p. *zir-duck.* زردک h. *gá-jir.* गाजर

(۱٤٥) اسغیداج الجصاصین IS-FEY-
DEJ'L'JUSSA-SEEN. Shell lime.
कली h. *kullee.* آهک صدف p. *á-huck fud-ef.*

(۱٤٦) اسغیدولیون US-KEE-DOO-
LE-YOON. Winter cherry.

(۱٤۷) اسران ÁSS-RÁN. Milk curds.

(۱٤۸) آس بنکه ÁSS-BIN-KEH.
Myrtle.

(۱٤۹) اسکنده US-GUN DEH. अस्तनोद
An Indian plant.
It is heating, and ftimulant.

(۱۵۰) اسروره US-RÚ-REH. Indian
fpikenard.

v. *fem-bel ut teil.* سنبل الطیب

(۱۵۱) اسخارهرومی ISS-KHÁ-REH-
ROOMEE. A thorny grafs.

(۱۵۲) آس بری ÁSS BIR-REE. Wild
myrtle.

(۱۵۳) اشهوسا & اسهوسا USH-MOO-SA
and US-MOO-SA. A fpecies of
merow.

(۱۵٤) اشیاف مامیسا Á-SHEYÁF
MÁ-MY-SÁ. The juice of a fpecies
of poppy.

(۱۵۵) اشنازداود USH-NÁZ DÁ-
OUD Dry hyffop; *vide* زوفا *zoofá.*

(۱۵٦) اشترغار USH-TUR-GHÁR.
Camel's thiftle.

(۱۵۷) اشتلایوس ISH-TE-LÁ-YOOS
An aromatic bark.
v. *dár-fhee-fhán.* دارشیمشعان

(۱۵۸) اشراش ISH-RÁSS. A plant, of
which is made a very ftrong glue.
सनेस h. *fir-eys.* سریشم p. *fir-ey-fhem.*

(۱۵۹) اشخیص ISH-KHEES. A fpecies of mezereon.

(۱٦۰) اشق USHUCK. Gum ammoniac.
صبغ

صمغ طراتيث   صمغ بل شبرين

p. *fe-mugh te-rá-tees*, and *fe-mugh bil fhe-reen.*

(161) اشقاقل ISH-KÁ-KUL. Wild carrot.

(162) اشكيل چشم USH-KYL CHESH UM. A fpecies of bramble.

v. *owfuj.*   عوسج

(163) اشنان USH-NÁN. Glaffwort.

चूक & चुनकशयः   غاسول

h. *chook.* & *chu-buck fhow-yeh.* p. *ghá-ful,*

qu. hot and dry 2. *prop* detergent and cauftic. *eh.* the beft grows at Bark near Cufah, and is of a light green. *d.* half a direm. *cor.* poppy. *fuc.* foap.

(164) آش بچكان ÁSH BUTCHE GÁN. Caftor.

(165) اشنه USH-NEH. Mofs that grows in trees.

छरीला   دواله

h. *cheree-lá.*   p. *de-wá-leh.*

(166) اصل الهندبا USS'LÚL HIN-DU-BA. Root of fuccory.

(167) اصل العرطنيثا USS'LUL UR-TE-NY-SA. Root of arthenita, or fowbread.

بخور مريم

(168) اصل الغرب USS'LU'L GHERB. Root of the mountain pine.

qu. hot and dry 2.

(169) اصل القصب USS'LU'L KUS-SEB. Root of the reed.

qu. hot and dry 2.

(170) اصل الذرت USSUL'Z'ZURT. Root of a fpecies of millet.

p. *beykh jew-ár.*   بيخ جوار

qu. cold and dry. *prop.* narcotic.

(171) اصابع الغتيات Á-SÁBA-UL-FE-TÉ-YAT. Sweet bafil.

तुलसी   انكشت كنيزكان

h. *tu'lfee.* p. *ungoofht kun-ee-zuck-án.*

(172) اصل الرازيانج USSUL'UR RA-ZEE-Á-NUJ. Root of a fpecies of anife.

सनकिजर   بيخ باديان

h. *fownf key jir.* p. *beykh bá-dy-án.*

(173) اصل اللغاح USSUL UL LOO-FAH. Mandrake root.

(174) اصل الجاوشير USSUL UL JE-WÁ-SHEER. Root of the opoponax tree.

p. *beykh gáwfheer.*   بيخ كاوشير

(175) اصل الكبر USSUL UL KUB-IR. Root of the caper bufh.   بيخ كبر

p. *bekyh kobir.*

(176)

(176) اصل المر USSUL 'L' MURR.

Root of the myrrh tree.

p. *beykh múrr.* بیخ مر

qu. hot and dry 2.

(177) اصل اللوز المر USSUL UL
LOWZ UL MURR. Root of the
bitter almond tree.

कनबेवादामकीजर بیخ بادام تلخ

h. *ke-ru-ey bádám key jir.* p. *beykh
bádám telkh.*

(178) اصابع صغر ÁSÁ-BÁ-SIFR. A
root. p. *kuf me-riem.* کف مریم

It is of a dark yellow colour, and accounted
good in curing the bite of any animal.

(179) اصابع هرمس ÁSÁ-BÁ HOOR-
MUS. Hermodactyls.

p. *foorinján.* کل سورنجان

(180) اصل السوس USSUL US' SOOS.
Liquorice root.

जीटीमद and मुलहठी بیخ مهک

h. *mooh-luttee,* and *jet-hee-mudh.* p.
beykh mé-huck.

(181) اصل الکرفس USSUL UL
KEREFS. Parſley root.

श्रजमुदकीजर بیخ کرفس

h. *uj-mood-key jir.* p. *beykh kerefs.*

(182) اصل السوسن الابیض USSUL

US' SO-SUN UL UBYEEZ. Root
of white lily.

p. *beykh ſo-ſun ſe-feid.* بیخ سوسن سفید

(183) اصل اللوف USSUL UL LOOF.

Root of dragonwort.

p. *beykh peel-gooſh.* بیخ پیلکوش

qu. hot and dry, 3.

(184) اصل الاصغ USSUL UL Á-SUF.

Root of the caper buſh; *vide* No. 175.

(185) اصطرک US-TE-RUCK. Storax.

qu. hot and dry. *cor.* coriander ſeed. *ſuc.*
coſtus.

(186) اصل التنبول USSUL UT TUM-
BOOL. Root of the betel plant.

तुलीजन بیخ پان

h. *ko-lin-jen.* p. *beykh pán.*

(187) اصل الغلغل USSUL UL FIL-
FIL. Root of the long pepper ſhrub.

(188) اصل النیل USSUL UL NEEL.

Root of *neel.*

p. *beykh hub ul neel.* بیخ حب النیل

The *neel* tree bears a purgative berry, called
in Arabic *hub ul neel.*

(189) اصل الراسن USSUL UL RÁ-
SUN. Root of elecampan e.

بیخ زنجبیل شامی

p. *beykh zunjé-beel ſhámee.*

qu. hot and dry, 2.

(190) اصل قنطافلون USSUL FIN-TÁ-FE-LOON. Root of cinquefoil.

p. *beykh punjungooſht.* بیخ پنج انشکت

qu. hot and dry, 2.

(191) اصطغين IS-TÉ-FEEN. Carrot.

(192) اصول الاربعه USSOOL UL ÁR-BÁ-Á. The four roots, *viz.* ſuccory, fennel, caper, and tamariſk.

(193) اصل الكثاه USS UL KUSS-ÁH. Parſley root.

(194) اصابع الغذاري ASÁ BA UL GHÉ-ZÁ-REE. A ſpecies of black grapes. कालीदाष انكورزيتوني

h. *ká-lee dúkh.* p. *uugoor zietoonee.*

qu. hot and dry.

(195) اصل المازريون USSUL 'L' MÁZ-RI-YOON. Mezereon root.

p. *beykh muſt-roo.* بیخ مستارو

qu. hot and dry, 3.

(196) اصل النيلوفرالهندي USSUL NEE-LU-FIR HINDEE. Root of water lily.

कवनकीजर h. *konwul key jir.*

بیخ نیلوفرهندي p. *beykh nee-lu-fir-hindee.*

(197) اصل السوسن الاسمان جوني USSUL US SO-SUN UL ASSMÁN JOO-NEE. Root of iris.

v. *jyrſá.* ایرسا

(198) اصل الخنثي USSUL'L'KHUN-SÁ. A glutinous root of a ſpecies of graſs. p. *beykh gee-há. ſé-rey-ſhum.*

بیخ کیاهسریشم

(199) اصل الانجدان الخراساني US-SUL'L'UN-JÉ-DAN-UL-KHORÁ-SÁNEE. Root of a ſpecies of thiſtle.

(200) اضراص الكلب UZRÁSS UL KELB. Polypody.

(201) اضموط UZMOOT. A kind of filbert.

(202) اطميسا UT-MEE-SÁ. Mugwort.

(203) اطاء E-TÁ-Á. The white poplar. *vide* 109.

(204) اطريغل IT-REE-FUL. General name for myrobalans.

(205) اطراف زيتون UT-RÁF ZIE-TOON. Olive branches.

p. *ſhákh-há zietoon.* شاخهاي زيتون

(206) اطريه UT-RY-EH. A kind of vermicelli.

M

सिवग्र

सिंबे

h. *seen-wi-ey.*   p. *hul-wa-iy rishteh.*   حلواي رشته

(207) اطباءالكبه UT-BÁ UL KEL-BEH. Sebestens.

(208) اظغارالطيب UZFÁR UT TEJB. Perfumed nails.

(209) اعين السراطين AI-YUN US SERÁTEEN. Seed of agnus castus. *vide* 35.

(210) اغبر UGBAR. A Collyrium.

It is composed of wormseed, tutty, and sugar candy.

(211) اغيرس Á-GHEE-RIS. Walnut. *vide* 46.

(212) اغيس Á-GHEES. One of the many names for agnus castus.

(213) اغرسطس UGHER-SE-TIS. A species of thistle.

v. *feel.* سيل   p. *beyd gee-á.* بيدكيا

(214) اغلقه UGH-LEE-KEH. Syrup of grapes, dates, &c.

p. *dúshab.* دوشاب

(215) اغالوجي ÁGHÁ-LOO-CHEE. Lignum aloes.

ॠगन   h. *ugir.*   p. *oud.* عود

(216) آفتاب پرست AF-TÁB PE-RUST. Worshipper of the sun.

This appellation is given to the sunflower, the neelufir, and the chameleon.

(217) افشرج UF-SHÚ-REJ. Expressed juice.

عصاره and افشرده

p. *uf-shoor-deh,* and *ussá-reh.*

(218) افرهنج UFRE-HUNJ. The herb curfuta.

p. *ku-shoos.* كشوث

(219) افكار UF-KÁR. Sneezewort.

नपिछेकनी h. *nuck chee-ké nee.*

(220) افرنجمشك ÁFRUNJ-MISHK. A species of sweet basil.

तुलसी   بالنكوي خورد

h. *túlsee.*   p. *bá-lun-goo-ee-khoord.*

qu. hot and dry, 2.   *cor.* violets.   *fuc.* cloves.

(221) اناسون ÁFÁ-SOON. Oil of radish.

मुनीकातिन   روغن ترب

h. *moo-lee ká teil.*   p. *roghen toorb.*

(222) افلاطون ÁFLÁ-TOON. Gum bdellium.

गूगुल h. *goo-gul.*   p. *mo-kul.* مقل

(223) انربيون E-FIR-BE-YOON. Euphorbium.

सिहंडकादुद फरنيون & شير درخت زقوم

h. *se-hoond ká doodh.*   p. *sheer derukht zuckoom.*   v. *fir-fi-yoon.*

It is the milky juice of a prickly plant, called *Zuckoom*, &c.

(224) افسنتين‎ UFSUNTEEN. Wormwood.

मसतारु‎ برنجاسف کوهي‎

h. *muf-tá-roo.*   p. *burunja-fif kouhee.*

  qu. hot and dry, 3. *prop.* deobftruent and purgative, and deftroying worms.

(225) افیلون‎ UFYLOON. Mountain wormfeed.

درمنه کوهي‎   p. *dir-me-neh kou-hee.*

(226) افیون‎ UF-YOON. Opium.

अफीम‎ شیر خشخاش‎

h. *uf-eem.*   p. *fheer khufh káfh.*

  qu. cold, 4. dry, 3.   *prop.* narcotic and fedative. *ch.* that which diffolves readily in water, and melts when expofed to the fun. *d.* The weight of a pea; for outward application, twice that quantity. *cor.* pepper, cinnamon, fagapenum, parfley feed, and caftor. *fuc.* three times the weight, of henbane feed, with one-third more of the fruit of mandrake.

(227) انتیمون‎ AFTEEMOON. Dodder of thyme.

अकासबिन‎   h. *ákafs beyl.*

(228) انادیه‎ AFÁ-DY-AH. Heating medicines, fuch as cloves, galangal, cinnamon, &c.

(229) انلنجه‎ IF-LUN-JEH. A feed, refembling muftard, but of a fragrant fmell.

p. *fe-lun-jeh.* فلنجه‎

It is chiefly u ed in perfumes.

(230) افعي‎ UF-IEY. Snake, in general.

साफ‎ h. *fámp.*   p. *mar:* مار‎

  qu. hot and dry, 4. *prop.* attenuant. *ch.* a female. *d.* of the flefh, three mifkáls. *cor.* Teriac or Venice treacle.

(231) اتاقیا‎ Á-KÁ-KYÁ. Acacia.

(232) اقلیمیا‎ EKLEE-MYA. The drofs of gold or filver.

  prop. drying. *cor.* oil of almonds.

(233) اتسوس‎ UK-SOOS. A fmall vifcous berry.

(234) اقط‎ U-KIT. Dried milk curds.

  qu. cold and dry.

(235) اقحوان‎ OKH-HYWÁN. Camomile flowers.

  p. *bábooneh gáw.* بابونه کاو‎

(236) اقویلاسمون رومي‎ ÁKOO-YEELÁ-SEMOON-ROOMEE. Balfam of Gilead.

  p. *roghen bulfán.* روغن بلسان‎

(237) اقارون‎ A-'KÁ-ROON. Sweet flag.

  p. *wuj.* وج‎

(238) اقطن یمني‎ UKTIN YEMENEE. A fpecies of vetch.

  p. *bé-noo-máfh.*

p. *bé-noo-máſh.* بنوماش

(239) اقومالي EKOO-MÁ-LEE. A mixture of honey and water.

(240) اقطي UK-TEE. The eider tree.

(241) اقطنالوقي UKTENÁ-LOO-KEE. A kind of white thorn.

दे माहा

h. *deh-má-há.* p. *búd-á-wird.* بادآورد

(242) اكتمكت UK-IT-MUCKIT. The eagle ſtone.

क नेजुवा

h. *kerun-jewá.* p. *kha-yeh eblees.* خايهابليس

Suppoſed to aſſiſt women in labour.

(243) اكشوث UKH-SHOOS. A ſpecies of dodder.

(244) اكمج UK-UJ. The medlar.

(245) اكر IG-IR. Sweet-ſcented flag.

(246) اكرفس UK-REFS. Parſley. v. *kerefs.* كرفس

(247) اكروفس UK-RU-FÚS. Walnut. p. *jowz-roomee.* جوزرومي

(248) آك AG. Name of a milky tree.

श्राग

a. *ſhejer úſhir.* شجرعشر

(249) اكروهك UK-ROO-HUCK. Sarcocolla; *vide No.*

(250) اكليلالملك EKLEEL'UL ME-LIC. Melilot.

श्रमपरक

h. *aſ-pe-ruck.* p. *gee-áh ky-ſir,* alſo *ze-reer.* vide 141. كياةقيصر زرير

(251) اكليلاهوض EKLEEL AH-WUZ. Seed of an Indian plant.

श्रतंगनकिबीज h. *u-tun-gun kay beedj.*

(252) آكويزان UK-MOO-YE-ZAN. A ſpecies of pea.

(253) آكارغون ÁKA-REE-KOON. Stone of the wild olive.

(254) اكلنغسه U-KEIL NEFSEH. Euphorbiʊm.

v. *fir-fy-oon.* فرفيون

(255) اكاهولي AKÁ HOO-LEE. An Indian plant.

श्राकाठुली

It is uſed in the caſe of the gonorrhœa.

(256) السا ULSA. A ſpecies of aniſeed.

(257) الب IL-IB. Aloes; *vide* 34.

(258) الوج Á-LOOJ. A plant, con-ſidered as an antidote.

p. *gíz-ruck.* كازرک

(259) السنةالعصافير UL-SINETUL ÁSÁ-

ÁSÁ-FEER. Sparrow's tongue, a feed.

इ दरजब لسان العصافبر اهر

h. *inderjoe.* a. *liſſán us áſá-feer.* p. *áhir.*

(260) الماس UL-MÁSS. Diamond.

हिरा h. *kee-rá.* p. *máſs.* ماس

(261) البانيس UL-BÁ-NEES. A

pot-herb. सांग चौलये h. *ſág chowlie.*

(262) البطوط ELIB-TOOT. A ſpe-

cies of creeper.

(263) الطارومي UL-UT-ROOMEE.

A ſpecies of mint. p. *ſec-ſubr.* سيسبر

(264) الانيون UL-Á--NEE-YOON.

Elecampane.

(265) اليبو UL-YOU. Adam's fig;

vide. 320.

(266) اليبه UL-YE-ÁH. Tail of the

Perſian ſheep.

दंबिके पुंछ دم دنبه

h. *dumbeyh key poontch.* p. *dúm dúmbeh.*

qu. hot and moiſt. *prop.* emollient.

(267) اله É-LÚK. The eagle.

p. *o-káb.* عقاب

(268) الاطبني A-LÁ-TEE-NEE.

Fluellin.

(269) الا يچي E-LA-IY-CHEE.

इलाची Cardamum ſeed.

(270) السي ULSEE. आलसी

Linſeed.

(271) امرا ÁM-RÁ. अम्रन An In-

dian fruit, in ſhape reſembling the

mangoe.

(272) املبينت ÁMUL BEYNT.

अमलबिंत An Indian fruit.

(273) آملج ÁM-LUJ. Emblic my-

robalans.

आंवरा h. *aunwerá.* p. *á-mu-leh.* أمله

(274) امرود UMROOD. Pear·

p. *náſhpátee.* ناشپاتي

(275) اموس Á-MOOS. Biſhop's

weed, ammi.

(276) امعاءالارض Á-MÁÁ UL URZ.

Earthworm.

(277) امعاسين U-MÁ-SEEN. Juice

of grapes.

दाखकापानी آبغوره انكور

h. *dakh káy pá-nee.* p. *áb ghowrá ungoor.*

(278) امامون A-MA-MOON.

Amomum.

(279) امغيلان UM GHEELÁN. The

gum-arabic tree. *vide* 414.

prop. aftringent., and drying. *d. ad libitum.*
cor. violets.

(280) انغطينا UN-FÉ-TEE-NÁ. *fy.*
Wild rofe.

(281) اناركيوا Á-NAR-GEE-WÁ.
Poppy.

(282) انساسا UN-SÁ-SÁ. Raifins.

(283) انجسا UN-JEY-SÁ. A fpecies
of buglofs.   v. p. *fhunkár.* شنكار

(284) انقرديا UN-KIR-DYÁ. Anacardium.

(285) انوميا UN-OO-MY-Á
Anemone.

(286) انطونيا UN-TOO-NY-Á.
Endive.

(287) انتلهسودا UN-TE-LEH-
SOWDÁ. Zedoary.   *vide.* 412.

(288) انكورشغا UNGOOR SHÉ-FA.
A fpecies of nightfhade.

(289) انب UN-UB. The egg plant.
vide 382.

(290) انزروت UNZEROOT.
Sarcocolla.   p. *kun-ju-deh.* كنجده

(291) انجوج UNJOOJ.   Lignum
alœs. *vide* 216.

(292) انكور UNGOOR. Grapes.
दाख: h. *dák,h.*

(293) انجير UNJEER.   Fig.
a. *teen.*   تين

(294) انبرباريس UN-BER-BÁ-REES.
Barberries.

(295) انجباررومي UN-JE-BÁR
ROOMEE.   A plant growing on the
banks of the Euphrates, ufed in ftop-
ping hemorrhages.

(296) اندروطاقس UNDRYO-TÁ-
KIS. a fpecies of vetch.

(297) اناعيلس UNÁ-EEY-LUS.
Marjoram.

(298) انغاق UNFÁK.   Olive oil.
p. *roghen zietoon.*   روغنزيتون

(299) انجرك UNJERUCK. Marjoram.

(300) انجكك UNJOO-KUCK.
A fpecies of grain refembling pear-feed

(301) آنك Á-NUK.   Lead.

(302) انجل UNJIL.   Marfh-mallows.

(303) انغغونرومي UN-FU-KÚN-
ROOMEE. A fpecies of rofe without
fmell.

सदागुलाब   كل پياده
h. *fud-*

h. *ſud-á gooláb.*   p. *gool pe-yá deh.*

(304) انيسون   Á-NEE-SOON.
Aniſeed.

सोन्फ   راز ياندرومي
h. *ſownf.*   p. *rá-zy-á-neh roomee.*

(305) انجدان   UN-JU-DAN. The
aſafœtida plant.

हिंगकारोख   درخت‌انكوزه
h. *hing ká rookͪh.*   p. *dirukht un-goo-zeh.*

qu. hot and dry, 3. *prop.* deobſtruent, attenuant, and diaphoretic. *ch.* white. *d.* one direm.
cor. vinegar. *ſuc.* the root thereof.

(306) اندراين   IN-DE-RÁ-YEN.
इंदरायन The fruit of the coloquintida
plant. p. *hunzil.*   حنظل

(307) انجن UNJUN. अंजन Collyrium in general.

(308) اندروخورون   UNDEROO-
KHU-ROON.   A weed that grows
amongſt wheat and barley, the ſeed of
which is red, and very bitter.

(309) اندرجو INDIR-JOW. इंदरजोब
Sparrow's tongue.   A ſeed.   *vide* 261.
p. *liſſán ul us-á-feer.*   لسان‌العصافير

(310) انجيده UN-JEE-DEH.   Wild
leek.

(311) انغخه UN-FÉ-KEH.   Rennet

in general.   चुमन: پنيرمايه
h. *chuſtah.*   p. *pé-neer-má-yeh.*

qu. hot and dry, 2. *prop.* attenuant and deobſtruent. *ch.* that which has been ſqueezed quite
dry. *cor.* honey.

(312) انغخةالارنب   UN-FÉ KÉTUL
URNEB. Rennet of a hare.

پنيرمايه‌خرکوش
p. *pé-neer-má-yeh khurgooſh.*

(313) انغخةالغرس   UNFÉ KÉTÚL
FERES.   Rennet of a horſe.

(314) انغخةالخشف   UNFÉ KÉ-
T'UL KHI-SHIF. Rennet of a male kid
of a mountain-goat, that is a firſtling.

(315) انغخةالجبل   UN-FÉ-KÉ-TÚL
JÉ-MÉL.   Rennet of a camel.

(316) انغخةالعجل   UN-FE-KE-
T'UL E-JIL.   Rennet of a calf.

(317) انقطريون   IN-KIT-REE-
YOON.   Amber.

(318) انكبيين UN-GU-BEEN. Honey.

(319) انجره ١ UN-JE-REH.   Nettle.
बिटगन   کزنه
h *á-tun-gen.*   p. *guz-neh.*

(320) انجيردشتي   INJEER DESH-
TEE. Adam's fig.   *vide* 265.

v. *in-*

v. *injeer Adém.* انجبرادم

(321) انبوت‌الراعي UMBOOT'TR-RA-IY. A fpecies of Houfe-leek.

(322) انبوت‌ملكي UMBOOT MUL-E-KEE. The amaranth.

(323) انكبه UN-KÚ MEH. The inverted thorn.

(324) اناليغي‌رومي UN-Á-LEE-KEE-ROOMEE. Nettle.

(325) انبلي UMBLEE इमली Tamarind. p. *temr hindee.* تمرهندي

(326) اومادا OW-MÁ-DÁ. Expreffed juice of wild cucumber.

(327) اوكنج OW-KUNJ. Sebeftens.

(328) اوسپيد OWS-PEYD. A fpecies of water lily.

(329) اوذر OW-ZIR. Water. पानी h. *pá-nee.* a. *maá.* ماء p. *db.* آب

(330) اوز OWZ. Water-fowl. *vide* 6.

(331) اونانيس OW-NÁ-NEES. Pomegranate buds.
p. *fhé-goo-feh á-nár.* شكوفةانار

(332) اوشع OW-SHÁ The marten, or fable. p. *fé-moor.* سمور

(333) اوداساليون OW-DÁ-SÁ-LI-YOON. Wild Parfley.
p. *kerefs kou-hee.* كرفس‌كوهي

(334) اوقيمن OW-KY-MUN. Wild fweet bafil.

(335) اوقطاريون OW-KÉ-TÁ-RI-YOON. Hemp agrimony.

(336) اورمالبي OWR-MÁ-LEE. Juice refembling honey, obtained from a certain tree, whofe name is not mentioned.

(337) اونومالي OW-NOO MÁ-LEE. A mixture of honey and wine.
p. *fhé ráb wu afful.* شراب‌وعسل

(338) اهليلج‌اسود AH-LEE-LUJ US-WUD. Black myrobalans.
जंगीहर هليله‌سياه
h. *zun-gee hár.* p. *he-lee-leh fee-áh.*
qu. cold 1, dry 2. *prop.* eathartic. *ch.* black. *d* of the fkins 1 or 2 direms; in decoction 7 to 10 direms. *cor.* honey. *fuc.* chebulic myrobalans.

(339) اهليلج‌اصفر AH-LEE-LUJ ASFIR. Yellow myrobalans.
हरतकी هليله‌زرد
h. *hirtuckee.* p. *hé-lee-leh zird.*
qu. cold 1, dry 2.—*prop.* cholagoga and tonic.—*ch.* plump. *d.* of the fkins as far as 5 direms; in decoction from 7 to 20 direms. *cor.* fugar-candy or manna, with jujubes.

(340) اهلال‌القسط AH-LÁL UL KOUST. A fpecies of fweet bafil.

(341) اهک Á-HUCK. Lime.

चुना   h. *choo-ná.*

(342) اهلیلج کابلي AH-LEE-LUJ CÁ-BULEE. Chebulic myrobalans.

अंबयाहर   هليله کلان

h.*umbe-á-hér.*   p. *he-lee-leh kelán.*

> qu. cold and dry. *prop.* melanagoga. *ch.* large and plump, and that will sink in water. *d.* 5 to 10 direms. *cor.* honey. *suc.* black myrobalans.

(343) IYR-SÁ. Root of blue iris.

> qu. hot and dry. *prop.* suppurative, and deobstruent. *ch.* black and hard, full of knots, and fragrant. *d.* 2 direms. *cor.* honey.

(344) ايلوا EY-LEW-Á. ऐलवा Aloes.   p. *syb-ir.* صبر

(345) اینکر IN-GUR. ऐंगुर Vermilion.   p. *shin-girf.* شنکرف

(346) ايدعرومي IY-DÁ-ROO-MEE. Dragon's blood.

(347) ايل EE-YUL. The mountain cow.   p. *gau kou-hee.* کاوکوهي

(348) ايهقان IY-KU-KÁN. A species of lupin.

(349) ابرسون EER-SOON. Talc; *vide* 16.

(350) ايرون IY ROON. Yellow orpiment. p. *gow-gird zird.* کوکرد زرد

(351) ايرن IY-RUN. Milk curds. p. *dowgh.* دوغ

(352) ايغاقين EY-KÁ-KEIN. Lignum aloes.   p. *owd.* عود

(353) ابرقان EER-KÁN. A species of privet.   p. *henna.* حنا

(354) ايرفيون EER-FI-YOON. The violet.

ب

(355) باقلا BÁ-KÉ-LÁ. A species of bean.

> qu. cold and dry, 2. *prop.* astringent.

(356) بالا BÁLÁ. बाला also KEN-DUL. कंदुल An odoriferous grass.

> It is used for tents and doors in the hot season, and being kept wet, the wind in passing through is cooled from 120 to 76 degrees.

(357) باجرا BÁJ-RA. बाजरा A species of grain used for food

(358) بانسا BANSA. बांसा also A-RUSÁ. अरुसा An Indian plant.

(359) پانڑا PÁD-RÁ. पाउरा also PÁ-DUL. पाउल Flower of an Indian tree.

> It is used as a perfume.

O

(360) پات PÁT. पात Raw filk, *vide* 20.

(361) باردست BÁR-DUST. Ebony. *vide* 12.

(362) بادنج BÁDNUJ. Cocoanut.

(363) بابونج BÁBOONUJ. Camomile flower.

    qu. hot and dry. *prop.* attenuant, deobftruent, and difcutient. *ch.* large yellow flower. *d.* a pugil. *cor.* honey, or oil of rofes. *fuc.* milolet, or mugwort.

(364) بادروج BÁD-ROOJ. A fpecies of fweet bafil.

ज़ंगलीतोलसी   تره خراساني

h. *junglee tulfee.* p. *tur-eh khorájánee.*

    qu. hot and dry. *prop.* deobftruent, cordial, ftyptic. *ch.* frefh and pungent. *d.* of the feed 2 direms. *fuc.* tulfee.

(365) باداورد BÁ-DÁ-WÚRD. A prickly fhrub.

जओनवाफा   شوكةالبيضا

h. *jownwáfa* a. *fhowkt ul'-by-zá.*

(366) بارود BÁ-RUD. Fixed alkali falt, natron. *vide* 129.

(367) باراهيكند BÁRA-HY-KUND. बाराहिकंद An Indian plant.

    qu. hot and dry 1. *prop.* drying. *ch.* frefh, white leaves. *d.* one direm and a half. *cor.* wormwood. *fuc.* fumitory.

(368) بارزد BÁR-ZUD. Galbanum.

बरीज   بيزد   ته

h. *bir-ee-já.* p. *beer-zud.* v. *kunneh.*

    qu. hot 3, dry 2. *ch.* foft, and yellow, like honey; pungent. *cor.* gum ammoniac. *fuc.* fagapenum.

(369) پاكهان بهيد PÁ-KHEN-BHIED. पाषानबिद Gentian.

(370) پاكر PÁKIR पाकर An Indian fruit tree.

(371) پادزهر PÁD-ZEHR. Bezoar.

ज़हरमुहर: پاي زهر

h. *zehr-moh-rir.* p. *pá-iy zehr.*

(372) بابوسر BÁ-BOO-SIR. Adulterated camphor.

(373) بابسر BA-BE-SIR. Another name for fenna.

(374) بانس BÁNS. बांस Bamboo.
p. *ni-ee hin-dee.*   ني هندي

    qu. cold. *prop.* emollient.

(375) باروق BÁ-ROOK. Ceruffe of tin, or of lead.

(376) پالك PÁ-LÚCK. Spinnage. *vide* 121.

(377) باي برنك BÁ-IY BERENG. A grain refembling pepper.

    qu. hot and dry.

(378) بالنك BÁ-LUNG. A fpecies of citron, *vide* 7.

(378)

(379) بارتنك BAR-TUNG. Ribwort.

(380) بادام BÁ-DAM. Almond.

a. *lowz.* لوز

(381) پان PAN. पान Betel leaf.

p. *birg tumbowl.* برك تنبول

(38.) باذنجان BÁD-IN-JAN. The egg plant. बैगुन बहंटा

h. *byn-gun* and *báhn-ta.*

(383) بان BÁN. The Perſian lilac.

बकायन h. *buck-á'yin.*

(384) بارسطاربون BÁR-IS-TAR-YOON. Vervain.

(385) باديان BÁDEE-YAN. *p.* A ſpecies of aniſeed.

(386) بارو BÁROO, बारू alſo BÁ-LOO. बाल Sand. p. *reyg.* ريك a. *reml.* رمل

(38;) باتو BÁ-TOO. A purgative ſeed. v. *dund.* دند जमालगोटा *jemál gowtá.*

(388) بادرنجبويه BÁD RUNJ-BOO-YEH. A ſpecies of ſweet baſil.

h. *rám tulſee.*

(389) بالنكو BALUN-GOO. Another name for the above.

(390) بابوسه BÁ-BOO-SEH. The bud of any tree. कुन्दल h. *kown-pul.*

(391) بابله BA-BÚ-LEH. Liquid Storax.

(392) باخه BÁ-KHEH. The tortoiſe.

कि छुआ سنك پشت

h. *kutch-he-wá.* p. *ſung púſht.*

(393) بابونه BABOONEH. Camomile flowers.

(394) باقلاقبطي BÁ-KE-LA KIP-TEE. Egyptian lupin.

(395) باقلامصري BÁ-KÉ-LA MIS-REE. The ſame.

(396) باجي BAJEE. *h.* Nitre. *vide* 9.

(397) باباري BÁ-BÁ-REE. *ſy.* Black pepper.

(398) بارهي BÁR-HEE, alſo NEER-BISSEE. Zedoary. बा नहि & नरबसी v. *jedwar.* جدوار

(399) ببغا BUB-GHÁ. *a.* A parrot. h. *tow-tá,* and *ſew-a.* p. *too-tee.* طوطي

(400) ببول BA-BOOL. The gum arabic tree. p. *mugheelán.* مغيلان

(401) پتپاپرا PIT-PÁP-RÁ. पितपापरा Fumitory.

p. *ſháhtereh.* شاهتره

(402) پنجیا PUT-JE-ÁY. पतजेया An Indian tree.

(403) بتهوا BUT-HEW-A. नतवा Orach.

(404)

(404) بجورا BE-JEW-RÁ. *h.*

Citron. *vide* 30.

(405) بجريهانک BUJ-JIR BHANG.

ञोग Tobacco. *v. tumbá-coo.* تنباكو

qu. hot and dry 4. *prop.* narcotic, and de-obstruent. *cor.* milk. In the appendix is an account when this plant was brought into Hindostan.

(406) بجم BOOJM. Fruit of the tamarisk.

मायैन ثمرةالطرفا كزمازو

h. ma·een *p. guz-má-zoo.* *a. sumrut ul-turfeh.*

(407) بخورمريم BÉ-KHOOR MI-RIEM. Sowbread.

v. shejereh miriem. شجرهمريم

(408) بدليون BUD-LEE-YOON. *sy.* Bdellium.

गुग्गल *h. goo-gul.* مقل *v. mo-kul.*

(409) پدلون PUD-LOON. पटलौन Salt of bitumen.

p. nemuck see-yah. نمكسياه

(410) برهتنيا BE-REH-TYÁ. बरहनेया also BUDDES KUT-Á-IY बुद्दीकटयै An Indian prickly shrub.

(411) بر BURR. Wheat.

गिहूं *h. geehoon.* *p. gundum.* كندم

(412) بر BIR. बर An Indian fruit-tree.

a. zát uz-ze-wánib. ذاةالذوانب

(413) برنجاسف BIR-UN-JA-SIF.

Mugwort. गंदमार *h. gund-már.*

ch. yellow. *cor.* aniseed.

(414) برقوق BIR-KOOK. Apricot.

घोबानी مشمش

h. khoobá-nee. *p. mishmish.*

(415) برواق BIR-WAK. The herb asphodel.

v. gee-á-sir-eys. كياهسريس

(416) برنجمشك BERUNJ-MISHK.

A species of sweet basil. *vide* 364 & 388.

(417) بربال BIR-BÁL. बरबाल

Coral. मूंगा مرجان بسد

h. moongá. *a. bussed.* *p. mirján.*

(418) برغول BIR-GHOWL. Wheat coarsely ground.

p. de-lee-deh gundum. دليدهكندم

(419) برتوم BIRTOOM. Dates well dried.

p. khurmá-iy heeroon. خرماي هيرون

(420) پرشوم PIR-SHOOM. The reed.

(421) برم BURUM. Buds of the gum arabic tree.

(422) بردوسلام BURD-WU-SA-LAM. Ribwort. *vide* 379.

p. wer-

p. *weruck bartung.* ورق بارتنك

(423) برسن BEER-SOON. Cotton.

रूई h. *rew-ey.* p. *poombeh.* پنبه

(424) پرسیاوشان PIR-SY-OW-SHÁN. Maiden hair.

राजहंस h. *raj hunſs..*

qu. hot and dry. ch. dark red ſtalks with green leaves. d. three to ten direms. ſuc. violets, and root of liquorice.

(425) برنان BIR-NÁN. बरनान

A tree growing in Ajmeer, uſed for making roſaries.

(426) پرشیان دارو PIR-SHE-YÁN DA-ROO. A pot-herb, of a red colour.

qu. cold, and dry. ſuc. nightſhade, or ribwort.

(427) برنج کابلي BIR-UNJ CABU-LEE. A grain reſembling poppy.

बाबरंग h. *bá-iy be-rung.* برنك p. *berung.*

qu. hot and dry. prop. aſtringent, and *anthelmintic.* ch. ſmall, reddiſh. d. three to ten direms with new milk. cor. gum tragacanth. ſuc. Turkiſh lupins.

(428) بردي BIR-DEE. The Egyptian papyrus. पतीरा تك

h. *put-ee-rá.* p. *tuck.*

(429) برطانیغي BIR-TÉ-NEY-KEE. The flower called cockſcomb.

BUZIR KE-TOO-NÁ. (430) بزرقطونا

Seed of fleawort. p. *uſ-pé-ghool.* اسپغول

qu. cold and moiſt. prop. diſcutient. ch. large, of a dark red, and that will ſink in water. d. two to three direms. cor. gum tragacanth. ſuc. quince feed

(431) بزرالقثا BUZIR UL KIS-Á.

Seed of a ſpecies of cucumber.

ककरी के बीज h. *kuckree key beej.* p. *tokhem khyar-zeh.* نخم خیارزه

qu. cold and moiſt. ch. large, and full. cor. oxymel. ſuc. cucumber feed.

(432) بزرالهندبا BUZIR UL HIN-DU-BÁ. Endive feed.

p. *tokhem káſ-nee.* نخم کاسني

qu. temperate. ch. cultivated, freſh, and full. d. two to three direms. ſuc. oxymel.

(433) بزریقلةالحمقا BUZIR BUCK LET UL HÚKÉ MÁ. Purſlain feed.

लोनेया के बीज h. *loonyá key beej.* p. *tokhem túruck,* نخم تورک وخرنه and *kherefeh.*

(434) بزرالسداب BUZIR US SUD-ÁB. Seed of rue.

qu. hot and dry. ch. black and large. d. one to two direms. ſuc. gum tragacanth.

(435) بزرالغنب BUZ-IR-UL KUN-NEB Hemp feed.

सं के बीज

संने बीज

تخم بنك

h. *fun key beej.*   p. *tokhem bung.*

(436) بزرالكرنب BUZ-IR-UL KIR-NUB. Cabbage-feed.

p. *tokhem kullum.*   تخم كلم

(437) بزرالشبت BUZR'US SHIB-BET. Fennel feed.

सुवै के बीज   h. *few-ay key beej.*

qu. hot and dry. prop emetic, d. two di-rems. cor. honey.

(438) بزرللغت BUZ-IR UL LUFT. Turnip feed.

p. *tokhem fhulghum.*   تخم شلغم

qu. hot and moift. ch. large, and red. d. two direms. cor. melon feed.

(439) بزرالغنجنكشت BUZ-IR-UL FUNJUNGOOSHT. Seed of the agnus caftus.

संनालुके बीज   h. *fumb ha loo key beej.*

qu. hot and dry. ch. large. d. two direms. cor. milk.

(440) بزرالكشوث BUZ-IR-UL KE-SHOOS. Seed of the plant cufcute.

अमरबिद के बीज   um-er beyl key beej.

d. two direms. cor. honey. fuc. endive feed.

(441) بزرالكراث BUZ-IR-UL KUR-RASS. p. *tokhem gundná.* تخم كندنا

(442) بزرالبنج EUZ-IR-UL BUNJ. Black henbane-feed. vide 42.

ch. black prop. aftringent, and ftyptic. d. one to two dangs. cor. honey. fuc. opium.

(443) بزرالكاكنج BUZ-IR UL KAK-NEJ. Seed of the Winter cherry.

تخم عروسك در پرده

p. *tokhem u-roofuck dir pirdeh.*

(444) بزرالرازيانج BUZ-IR-UL RÁ-ZI-YÁ-NEJ. A fpecies of anifeed.

मोनफ   تخم باديان

h. *fownf.*   p. *tokhem badyán.*

(445) بزرالبطيخ BUZ-IR-UL BE-TEEKH. Mufk-melon feed.

p. *tokhem khirboozeh.*   تخم خربزه

qu. hot and moift. prop. when dry it is emetic. d. two to five direms. cor. honey.

(446) بزرالاسفناح BUZ-IR UL IS-FANAJ. Spinnage feed. vide 121.

(447) بزرالرشاد BUZ-IR UL RE-SHÁD. Seed of garden creffes.

हालेम   تخم تره تيزك

h. *he-lém.* p. *tokhem terreh tey-zuck.*

(448) بزرالقسد BUZ-IR-UL KUS-UD. Cucumber feed.

विश

बीर के बीज تخم خياربالنك

h. *kee ray key beej.* p. *tokem khyár bálung.*

بزرالورد (449) BUZ-IR UL WURD.

Roſe ſeed.

prop. aſtringent, and ſtyptic. *ch.* that of the Perſian roſe. *d.* 2 direms. *cor.* tragacanth.

(450) بزرالعصغر BUZ-IR UL US-FIR. Seed of ſafflower.

कुसुमकेबीज خسك دانه

h. *kuſoombh key beej.* p. *khuſ-uck dáneh.*

(451) بزباز BUZ-BAS. M cᵊ.

जबत्री بسباسه

h. *jaw-itree.* v. *biſ-bá-ſeh.*

(452) بزرالخس BUZ-IR-UL KHUSS. Lettuce ſeed.

p. *tokhem ká-hoo.* تخم کاهو

qu. cold and dry. *d.* one to two direms. *cor.* maſtich.

(453) بزرالاسقبينس BUZ-IR-BUL-Á-SE-KEES. Seed of garden creſſes. *vide* 450.

(454) بزرالحماض BUZ-IR-UL HU-MAZ. Sorrel ſeed.

चुके केबीज تخم ترشه

h. *chewká key beej.* p. *tokhem tu'rſheh.*

qu cold and dry. *ch.* of a reddiſh brown. *d.* two direms. *cor.* parſley ſeed, and aniſeed.

بزرالمط (455) BUZ-IR'UL MUT.

Seed of wild pomegranate.

p. *anardaneh deſhtee.* اناردشتي

بزرالسرمق (456) BUZ-IR UL SIR-MUC. Seed of orach.

ननविकेबीज تخم قطف

h. *but-hoo-á key beej.* p. *tokhem kitf.*

بزرالسلق (457) BUZ-IR UL SULK.

Beet ſeed.

p. *tokhem chukundir.* تخم چقندر

(458) بزاق BU-ZAK. Saliva.

राल लार لعاب دهن

h. *ral,* alſo *lár.* p. *lu-áb dehn.*

(459) بزرک BUZRUC. Linſeed.

p. *tokhem kut-án* تخم کتان *vide* 273. and 467.

(460) بزرالغجل BUZ-IR UL FUJL.

Radiſh ſeed.

मुली केबीज تخم ترب

h. *moolee key beej.* p. *tokhem toorb.*

qu. hot and dry. *prop.* emetic, and ſtimulent *d.* two direms. *cor.* coriander ſeed.

(461) بزرالسان الحمل BUZ-IR UL LISSAN UL HEML. Seed of Rib-wort. بارتنك p. *bartung.*

qu.

qu cold and dry.   *ch.* of a reddish brown.   *d.* three direms.   *cor.* honey.   *fuc.* forrel feed.

(462) بزرالبصل BUZ-IR-UL BUS-SUL.   *p. tokhem py-az.* تخم پياز

qu. hot and dry.   *d.* two direms.

(463) بزرالخمخم BUZ-IR UL KHOOMKHOOM.   Seed of wild pomegranate.   *vide* 458.

(464) بزرالكتان BUZ-IR-UL KUTÁN.   Linfeed.   *vide* 462.

(465) بزرالنمام BUZ-IR-UL-NÁMAN.   Seed of mother of thyme.

बरनानकेबीज   تخم سيسنبر

h. bernan key beej. p. tokhem fee-fumber.

ch. black.   *d.* three direms.   *cor.* gum tragacanth.   *fuc.* linfeed.

(466) بزرالهليون BUZ-IR UL HULYOON.

नागदोनकेबीज   تخم مارحوبه

h. nag-done.   p. tokhem már-chowbeh.

qu. hot and moift.   *d.* two direms.   *cor.* honey.

(467) بزرالريحان BUZ-IR UL RYHAN.   Sweet bafil feed.

तोलसीकेबीज   *h. tulfee key beej.*

qu. hot.   *prop.* aftringent.   *d.* one mifkál with cold water, or rofe water.   *cor.* fweet marjoram.

(468) بزرالمارزيون BUZ-IR UL MÁZRI-YOON.   Mezereon feed.

p. tokhem muft-ru. تخم مستارو

prop. emetic.

(469) بزرالرطبه BUZ-IR UL RUTBEH.   Seed of an odoriferous grafs.

p. tokhem afpift. تخم اسپست

qu. hot and moift.   *ch.* yellow.   *fuc.* turnip feed.

(470) بزرالخرفه BUZ-IR UL KIRFEH.   Purflain feed.

लोनेधाकेबीज   تخم تورك

h. loony-án key beej.   tokhem tu-ruck.

qu. cold, 3.   *d* in acute fevers, an infufion of five direms.   *cor.* fugar candy.   *fuc.* feed of fleawort.

(471) بزرالهوه BUZ-IR UL HEEWEH.   Seed of mallows.

p. toodree. تودري

(472) بزرالانجره BUZ-IR UL UNJEREH.   Nettle feed.

अरटंगेकेबीज   تخم كزنه

h. utungen key beej.   p. tokhem guzneh.

qu. hot and dry.   *d.* half a mifkál to three direms.   *fuc.* feed of creffes.

(473) بزرالكرفس البستاني BUZ-IR UL KEREFS UL BOSTÁNEE Garden parfley feed.   *vide* 38.

(474) بزرالخبازي بزرالخطمي BUZ-IR UL KHUBÁZE, and BUZ-IR UL KHII-

KHITMEE. Mallows, and marſh-mallows ſeed. *vide 471.*

ſuc. cucumber ſeed.

(475) بزرالرمان البري BUZ-IR UL RU-MAN UL BIR-REE. Seed of wild pomegranate.

(476) بزرالجزرالبستاني BUZ-IR UL JUZR'IL BOSTÁNEE. Garden carrot ſeed.

गाजर कैबीज h. *gá-jir key beej.* تخم زردک p. *tokhem zirduck.*

d. one direm.

(477) بزرالجزرالبري BUZ-IR UL JUZR'IL BIR-REE. Seed of wild carrot. تخم کزرصحراي

p. *tokhem guz-ir ſerá-iy.*

(478) بزرالحندقوقي BUZ-IR UL HUND-KOW-KEE. Seed of the lote tree.

ſuc. tares.

(479) بزرالرازبانج الرومي BUZ-IR UL RÁZEE-A-NEJ UL ROOMEE. Aniſeed. p. *aneeſoon.* انيسون

(480) پستا PISTÁ. पिस्ता Piſtachio nut. a. *fiſ-tuc.* فستق

(481) بستج BIS-TUJ. *a.* Frankincenſe.

p. *koonder.* كندر

(482) بستيناج رومي BUS-TEE-TÁJ. ROOMEE. A ſmall creeping plant.

गुख़्रु h. *gookehroo.* p. *khuſ-uck.* خسك

(483) بسفايج BUSFA-IJ. Polypody.

कंगाली h. *khungálee.*

(484) بسد BU-SUD. *a.* Coral. *vide 417.*

(485) بسر BU-SUR. Unripe dates.

(486) بستان افروز BOSTÁN UF-ROZE. The plant cockſcomb.

जटाधारी and कलगा تاجخروس h. *je-tá-dáh-ree,* and *kulgá.* v. *táj khe-roos.*

qu. cold and dry. *prop.* aſtringent. *ch.* that which has been dried in the ſhade. *d.* two to four direms, or of the ſeed one miſkal. *cor.* frank-incenſe. *ſuc.* ſorrel.

(487) پستان سك PISTÁN SUG. *p.* Sebeſtens.

लसुरा h. *lehſoorá.* v. *ſepiſtán.* سپستان

(488) پستجو PIST JOW. Barley meal. p. *árud j w.* اردجو

(489) بسبلسه BUS-BÁ-SEH. Mace. *vide 451.*

(490) بشبش BUSH BUSH. Leaves of the coloquintida plant.

Q

(491) بشترغ BUSH-TURUGH.
Melilot. *vide* 250.

(492) بصل الذيب BUSSUL ÚZ'
ZEEB. A species of wild onion.
.v. *bulboos.* بلبوس

(493) بصاق القمر BU-SÁK-UL
KUMR. The moon stone. Selenites.
v. a. *hejr ul kumr.* حجر القمر

(494) بصل الغار BUSSUL-UL-FÁR.
Squills. *vide* 139.

(495) بصل النرجس BUSSUL-UL-
NURJIS. Root of the narcissus.
qu. hot and dry. *d.* two miskals for an emetic.

(496) بصاق BUSÁK. Saliva.
qu. hot and moist. *prop.* suppurative and deobstruent. *ch.* fasting.

(497) بصل العنصل BUSSUL-UL-
UNSUL. Squill. *vide* 139.

(498) بصل BUSSUL. Onion.
पयाज h. *pee-áj.* p. *pee-yáz.* پياز
qu. hot and dry. *prop.* discutient and attenuant.
ch. white. *d.* of the seed two direms. *cor.*
vinegar.

(499) بطيخ BE-TEEKH. Musk
melon. बिरबुज:
h. *khir-boozá.* خربوزه p. *khir-boozeh.*
qu. hot and moist. *prop.* stimulant, diuretic,
and detergent: the skin is emetic.

(500) بط . BÚT. ـه Goose
हंस h. *huns.* p. *káz.* قاز

(501) بطم BOOTM. The turpentine tree.

(502) بطيخ زقي BE-TEEKH ZIC-
KEE. Water-melon.
तरबुज h. *turbooz.* p. *hindu-á-neh.* هندوانه
qu. cold and moist. *ch.* sweet and juicy.

(503) بعر BÁR Globular dung of
animals.
मगनी h. *mig-nee.* p. *pishkel.* پشكل
prop. These are used in cataplasms.

(504) بق BUCK. Gnat.
मछर h. *much-hér.* p. *push-eh.* پشه

(505) بغر BUCKIR. Ox, bull, or cow.
गाय & बैल کاو
h. *byln,* and *gow.* p. *gáw.*

(506) بقلة الحمقا BUCKLUT'UL
HU-ME-KÁ. Purslain.
लुनिया साग تورك
h. *loonyá ság.* p. *tooruck.*
qu. cold and moist. *prop.* narcotic. *ch.* broad
leaves. *cor.* parsley.

(507) بقلة الزهرا BUCKLÚTÚL ZEH-
RÁ. The same.

(508) بقلة الضب BUCKLUT ÚZ-
ZUB. A species of sweet basil.
p. *bá-*

p. *ba-lun-goo bir-ree.* بالنكوي بري

(509) بقلةالعدس BUCKLUT UL' UD-US. Calamint.

p. *powd-neh birree.* پودنه بري

(510) بقلةالخطاطيف BUCKLUT UL KHE-TA-TEEF. Celadine.

(511) بقلةالملك BUCK LUT UL MELIC. Fumitery.

(512) بقلةالغزال BUCK LUT UL GHEZAL. Dittany.

(513) بقلةالغارستم BUCK LUT 'UL FARISTUM. Balm.

p. *badrunj bu-yeh.* بادرنجبويه

(514) بقلةالخراسانيه BUCK LUT UL KHORASANYEH. Sorrel.

(515) بقلةالاترجيه BUCKLUT'UL' UT-RU-JY-EH. Balm.

(516) بقلةالبارده BUCKLUTUL BA-RE-DEH. Ivy.

p. *lublab.* لبلاب

(517) بقلةالذهبيه BUCKLUT 'UZ' ZEH-BI-YEH. Spinnage. *vide* 121.

(518) بقلةالمبارك BUCLUT UL MOBARIC, and بقلةاللينه BUCK LUT UL' LI-YE-NEH. Arabic names for Purslain.

(519) بقم BUCKUM. Redwood.

(520) بقيس BUCKUS. The box tree.

(521) بكبر BUCK-BIR. Cassia fistularis.

p. *khyar chember.* خيارچنبر

(522) بكاين BUCKA-YIN. ककायन The Persian lilac.

(523) پلاسپاپرا PALASSPAPRA. पलासपापरा Seed of an Indian tree, called *pelah. vide* 528.

v. ढाककेबीज *dhak key beej.*

(524) بليلج BE-LEY-LUJ. Belleric myrobalans.

बहिरा h. *be-hey-ra.* p. *be-ley-leh.* بليله *qu.* cold. *prop.* astringent, attenuant, and tonic. *ch.* yellow, and ripe. *d.* one to three direms. *cor.* honey. *suc.* emblic myrobalans.

(525) بلج BE-LUJ. Unripe dates. कचीखजूर غورهخرما h. *kutchee kehjoor.* p. *ghowreh khurma. qu.* cold and dry.

(526) بلادر BE-LA-DUR. Anacardium. निलावा h. *beh-la-wa. qu.* hot and dry 4. *prop.* cephalic. *ch.* black, thick, and full of juice. *d.* one and a half direms. *cor.* sesami oil.

(527) بلس BU-LUS. White fig. p. *injeer sefeid.* انجيرسفيد

(528)

(528) پلاس PELASS. पलास An Indian tree. ठाक h. v. *dhák*. p. *peleh* پله

(529) بلوط BELOOT. Acorn.

qu. cold and dry. *prop.* aftringent, and ftyptic.

(530) بلوط الارض BELOOT UL URZ. Gemander. p. *kemá-dry-oon* کمادریوس

(531) بلوط الملک BELOOT UL MELIC. The Oak.

p. *fháh beloot*. شاه بلوط

(532) پلنک مشک BE-LUNG-MISHK. A fpecies of fweet bafil.

(533) بلبوس BUL-BOOS. A fpecies of wild onion.

(534) بیل BAYL. बिल An Indian fruit.

qu. hot and dry. *p.* aftringent. *ch.* fweet.

(535) پلاس پیپل PELASSPILPIL. पलास पीपल An Indian tree.

(536) پلول PULWUL. पलवल An Indian pulfe.

(537) بلسن BULSUN. A fpecies of vetch. मसूर h. *mufoor*. p. *ud-us*. عدس

(538) بلسان BU-LÉ-SÁN. The balfam. Tree of Egypt.

qu. hot and dry. *prop.* of the balfam, attenu-

ant, and deobftruent. *d.* half a direm. *cor.* fandel wood. *fuc.* olive oil, and caffia lignia.

(539) پنجنکشت PUNJUNGOOSHT. The agnus caftus tree. संजालु h. *fumbháloo*.

(540) بنفسج BEHUSSEJ. Violet. बनुसा h. *benofá*. p. *benufsheh*. بنفشه

(541) بنج BUNJ. Black henbane feed.

(542) بندق BUNDOOK. Filbert. v. *findook*. فندق

(543) پنجه مریم PUNJEH MIRIEM. Sowbread. हाथा जूरी h. *hát há iooree*.

(544) بنطافلون PENTAFELOON. Cinquefoil.

(545) بن BUN. Coffee. p. *tokhem keweh*. تخم قهوه

(546) بنس لوچن BUNS-LOW-CHUN. बंसलुचन Sugar of bamboo. p. *tub-fheer*. طباشیر

(547) بن کیهون BUN-GEY-HOON. बनगिहौं Wild wheat.

(548) پنداالو PIND-A-LOO. पंडालो An Indian efculent root.

(549) بنتومه BUN-TOO-MEH. A fpecies of dodder. आकासबेल h. *ákáfs beyl*.

(550) پنبه دانه PUMBEH DA-NEH.

Cot-

Cotton feed. बिनूला h. *bé-now-lá.*

(551) بندق هندي BUNDOOK HINDEE. An Indian nut.

रीठा h. *reetha.*

qu. hot and dry. *d.* twenty mifkals of the oil.

(552) بنج دشتي BUNJ DESHTEE. The thorn apple.

v. *jowz maiffil.* جوزمائل

(553) بوصير BOW SEER. Mullein.

(554) بورق BOORUC. Borax.

मुहागा تنكار بوره

h. *fow-há-gá.* p. *tinkar.* v. *booreh.*

qu. hot and dry. *prop.* detergent, cauftic, and emetic. *ch.* white, from Armenia. *d.* in clyf-ters, from one to two direms. *cor.* gum arabic: *fuc.* bitter falt.

(555) بوم BOOM. *p.* The owl.

उल्लू h. *u-loo.*

(556) بوزيدان BOO-ZY-DÁN. A thick, white root, about four inches long.

qu. hot and dry. *prop.* attenuant. *ch.* thick, white, and ftriped. *d.* one to two direms. *cor.* honey.

(557) بوقلمون BOO-KE-LEE-MOON. The chameleon. *vide* 136.

(558) پوپو POOPOO. *p.* The lap-wing. *a. hud-hud.* هدهد

(559) پودنه POWDENEH. Garden mint.

(560) بوره ارمني BOOREH URME-NY. Borax. *vide* 554.

(561) بول BOWL. Urine. *fhifheh* شاشه

(562) پوش دربندي POSH DER-BENDEE. A plant growing in Der-bend, which the natives bruife, and form into little bougies, and ufe as an eye-falve.

(563) پوي POW-EY. पूय A plant, which has tendrils like the vine, and bears a fruit refembling fox's grapes.

(564) بولسري BOWL-SIR-EE. बोलसरी An Indian tree, whofe fruit is a remedy for the toothach.

The flower has a pungency, which is increafed by being dried.

(565) بهيرا BE-HEY-RÁ. बहेरा Belleric myrobalan.

(566) پهلسا PHULSÁ. फालसा An Indian fruit.

(567) بهرامج BEH-RA-MUJ. A fpe-cies of willow.

p. *beid mufhk.* بيدمشك

(568) بهارامرود BEHAR UMROOD.

R Pear-

Pear blossoms. p. *gool umrood.* كل امرود
prop. cephalic.

(569) بهوجپتر BHOWJ-PUTTER.
नोऊपत्र The bark of a tree, which is used in Cashmeer for writing, instead of paper.

(570) بهانک BHANG. नांग A species of hemp.

The leaves are narcotic and aphrodisiac.

(571) بهرام and بهرمان BEHRAM, and BEHR-MAN. *p.* Seed of bastard saffron.

(572) پهکرمول PHO-KIR-MOOL.
An Indian root. फकरमूल

(573) بهمن BEH-MUN. A Persian root.

It is somewhat like a carrot, but is hard, crooked, rough, and pungent. There are two species, white, and red. Both are deobstruent and also accounted restorative.

(574) بهاربه BEHÁR BEH. Quince blossoms. *p. gool ab-ee.* كل آبي
prop. chephalic.

(575) پهتکري PHIT-KERRY.
फिटकरी Alum. *p. shub yemenee.*

(576) بینت BEYNT. बिंत Rattan.
p. kayz-ran. خيزران

(577) بیرزد BEER-ZUD. Galbanum.
बरिंजा *h. bir-ee-ja.*

(578) بیدانجیر BEID INJEER. The palma christi. *vide* 84.

(579) پیار PEE-YAR पेयार An Indian acid fruit, the seed of which is called *chorowngee.*

(580) بیر BEIR. बिर A species of plum. *p. konar.* كنار
qu. cold and dry.

(581) پیپلامور PEEPLÁMOOL.
पीपला मूल Root of the long pepper bush.

(582) بیخ سوس BEYKH SOOS. Liquorice root. *vide* 180.

(583) بیش BEESH. A poisonous root, brought from China.

(584) بیض BYZ. Egg in general. *p. tokh-m em janwar.* تخم جانور *h. unda.* उंडा

(585) پیپل PEEPUL. पीपल Long pepper.
It is also one of the names of the banyan tree.

(586) بیل BAIL. बिल An Indian fruit, containing in a hard sheil a pulp somewhat resembling the apricot in flavour.
qu. dry 3.

(587) پیتل PEETUL. पीतल Brass.
p. berunj. برنج

(588)

(588) پیلو PEELOO. पीलु The toothpick tree. *vide* 90.

(589) پینو PEENOO. Dried milk curds. *v. keroot.* قروت

(590) بیخ شانه دشتی BEHK SHÁNEH DESHTEE. Root of the comb tree. कंगनी के जर *h. kunghnee key jir.*

(591) بیخ چوچي BEYKH CHOO-CHEE. The leech root.

चुची के जर *h. choochee key jir,* and जों क की जर *jownk key jir.*

It is fo called, becaufe the fruit of this plant fticks like a leech.

ت

(592) تانبا TÁMBÁ तानबा Copper. p. *mifs.* مس

(593) تامر TÁ-MIR. The flower of forrel. चुके के फूल كل حماص *h. chooká key phool. p. gool hum-dz.*

(594) تانبول TÁM-BOOL. Betel leaf. पान & नागबेल برك تنبول *h. pán,* and *nág-beyl. p. birg tumbowl.*

(595) تباشیر TEBÁ-SHEER. Sugar of Bamboo. *vide* 546.

(596) تبر TIBR. Gold. सोना *h. fowná. p.* زر *zir,* and *tillá.* طلا

(597) تبكان TIB-KÁN. Any thorn. कांटा *h. kán-tá.* p. *khár.* خار

(598) تبن مكه TIBN MUCKEH. Camel's hay. *vide* 63.

(599) تریک TIT-REEK. तन्रीक Sumach.

(600) تنلي TUTLEE. तेतली The leech plant. *vide* 592.

(601) تخ TUKH. Sefamé. Seed, after the oil has been expreffed. तल *h. khul. p. gun-já-reh.* كنجاره

(602) تخم TOKHEM. *p.* Seed, in general. बीज *h. beej. a. buzir.* بزر

(603) تذرج TE-ZURJ. Pheafant. p. *teedero.* تدرو

(604) تر پهلا TRI-PHÉ-LÁ. त्रे फला General name for three kinds of myro-

ba-

balans. *vide* 204.

(605) اترابصيدا TIR-ÁB-SYDÁ.
Sidonian earth.

(606) ترمرا TRI-MEE-RA. त्रिमरा
A purgative feed.

(607) ترب TOORB. *p.* Radifh.
मुली *h. moolee.*

(608) تربد TURBID. Turbith root.
निसबत *h. nif-wut,* and नागपत्तर
nágputter.

    prop. purgative. *ch.* China.

(609) ترمس TUR-MISS. Egyptian
lupin.

(610) ترابالهالك TU-RÁB-UL-
HÁLICK. Arfenic. संबोलखार
h. fumbool-khár. a. fum-ul-fár. سم الغار

(611) ترنجبين TUREN-JEE-BEEN.
A fpecies of manna, collected at Khore-
fan. from a thorny plant, called *khár
fhooter.*

    prop. mild purgative. *ch.* refembling man-
na, and which is brought from Nifhápoor. *d*
from feven to thirty direms. *cor.* tamarinds.

(612) تریاق روستایان TERIAC
ROWSTYÁN. Garlic.

(613) تریاق الحیته TERIAC UL

HIHYEH. A bezoer ftone, which is
found in the corner of the eye of a
mountain ox.

(614) تریاق TERIÁC. Treacle. An-
tidotes. of every kind against poifons.
p. pád-zeher. پادزهر

(615) تریاق ترکي TERIÁC TOOR-
KEE. Mummy. *v. moo-mee-yi.* مومیایي

(616) ترهني TREHUTEE. त्रेहुती
White kuth.
कठसफेद *v. kath fefeid.*

(617) ترابالقي TU-RÁB-UL-KIE.
The emetic earth, arfenick. *vide* 613.

(618) تشمیزج TUSH MEEZUJ. A
black fhining feed, refembling that of
quince. चाक्सू *h. chákfoo.*
p. chefhmuck. چشمك
    qu. hot and dry.

(619) تفاح TUFFÁH. Apple.
p feeb. سیب

(620) تفاح الارض TUFFAH UL
URZ. Camomile flowers.
v. bá-boneh. بابونه *vide* 363.

(621) تفاح الجن TUFFÁH UL GIN.
Fruit of the mandrake.

                    (622)

(622) تفاح بری TUFFÁH BIR-REE.
Medlar.　　v. zá-roor. زعرور

(623) تفاح ارمنی TUFFÁH URME-
NEE. Apricot. v. khoobánee. خوبانی

(624) تفاح پارسی TUFFAH PARSEE.
Peach.　　v. shuft-á-loo. شفتالو

(625) تکرک TÉ-GURG. Hailstone.
ओला h. owlá.　　p. jháleh. ژاله

(626) تل TIL. तिल Sefamé feed.

(627) تلسی TULSEE. तोलसी
Sweet bafil.

p. bádrunj boo-yáh. بادرنجبویه

(628) تلی TILLEE. तेली The
milt, or fpleen.　p. fe-poorz. سپرز

(629) تمساح TIM-SAH. Aligator.
मगरमच्छ h. mugur-mutch. p. nehung.
نهنگ

(630) تمر TEMR. Date.
खजूर h. kehjoor.　　p. khurmá. خرما

　　qu. hot and moift. prop. detergent, and reftora-
tive. fuc. raifins.

(631) تمتم TUMTUM Sumach.
v. fumác. سماق

(632) تمرهندی TEMR HINDEE.
Tamarind. vide 325.

(633) تنکار TINCAR. Tincal.
h. fo-há-gá. सुहागा

(634) تن TUN. तन A flower,
ufed for dying yellow.

(635) توبال الحدید TÚBÁL UL
HEDEED. Drofs of iron. p. cherk
áhun. چرک آهن h. lo-háy ká-keet.
लोहेकीट

(636) توتیای زرد TOO-TEE-A
ZIRD. The Bafrah ftone.
p. fung bufree. سنک بصری
qu. cold 1, dry 2. prop. drying ulcers.

(637) تون TOON. तून Flowers of
the agnus caftus tree.

(638) توت TOOT. Mulberry.

(639) توت وحشی TOOT WUSHEE.
Blackberry.　v. áleek. علیق and toot
feh gool. توت سه کل

(640) تودری TOWDREE.　Seed
of mallows.
　prop. deobftruent, and detergent.　ch. yellow
d. half a mifkal.

(641) توری TU-RI-EY. तोरई An
Indian pot-herb.

(642) تونبری TOOMBREE. तोंबरी
Two fpecies of gourd, one fweet, and
the other bitter.

S

(643)

(643) تین TEEN. Fig. p. *injeer*, الجبیر

prop. detergent, and suppurative.

(644) تیندو TEINDOO. हिंदु

Fruit of the ebony tree.

ث

─

(645) ثافسیا SÁ-FEE SÁ. *g.* Gum of wild rue.

prop. caustic.

(646) ثالسقیس SÁ-LIS-KEES. Babylonian cresses.

v. herf babilee. حرف بابلي

(647) ثدي SUD-EE. The dugs of any animal. *p. pistan.* پستان

h. चुच्ची *choochee,* and जुजीया *ju-jeeyá.*

(648) ثعلب SÁLEB. Fox.

h. लोंबरी *look hree,* and लाबरी *loombree.* *p. ro-báh.* روباه

(649) ثعام SÁ-AM. White worm-feed.

p. dirmeneh fefeid.

(650) ثغاریر SÁGHÁREER. A small

species of melon, very delicious.

h. केचरी *kutch-e-ree.* p. *dust-um-boo-yeh.* دستنبویه

(651) ثلج SULJ. Snow.

पाला h. *pá-lá.* p. *burf.* برف

(652) ثلج چینی SULJ CHEENEE. China snow, a soft white stone, used as a collyrium.

qu. cold and dry. *prop.* detergent. *d.* 2 dangs. *suc.* crab's eyes.

(653) ثوم SOOM. Garlic.

लःसुन h. *lehsun.* p. *feer.* سیر

qu. hot and dry, 4. *prop.* attenuant. *rh.* large cloves. *d.* 3 cloves. *cor.* acids, oils, and greafy food.

(654) ثیل SEEL. A species of thistle. *vide* 213.

ج چ

─

(655) چاب CHAP. चाब An Indian fruit tree.

(656) جاوشیر JÁ-WE-SHEER. Gum

opopanax. *p. gáwsheer.* گاوشیر

qu. hot and dry, 2. *prop.* deobstruent, attenuant, diaphoretic, and discutient. *ch.* of a saffron colour, easily dissolving in water. When

fresh

fresh taken from the tree it is white, but afterwards changes to yellow; the solution resembles milk. *d.* half a direm. *suc.* of sagapenum, twice the quantity.

(657) جارالنهر JÁR-UL-NEHR. A water plant. *v. seluck ul ma.* سلق الماء

It resembles the *nelusir*, and appears just above the surface of the water.

(658) جاورس JÁ-WÉRS. A species of millet.

qu. cold and dry. *prop.* astringent. *cor.* oil of sweet almonds.

(659) جاسوس JÁSUS. A species of white poppy. *p. khush-kásh zub-e-dee.* خشخاش زبدي

(660) جايپهل JÁ-I-PHUL जायफल Nutmeg. *p. jowz bew-á.* جوزبوا

(661) جامن JAMUM, जामुन and پهلندا PHÉLINDÁ. फलनदा Names of an Indian fruit, resembling black grapes; it has a large stone.

qu. dry. *prop.* astringent.

(662) چاكسو CHÁK-SU. चाकसू A black seed, resembling that of quince.

(663) جامسه JÁ-ME-SEH. A species of lupin.

(664) جالي JÁ-LEE. The tooth-prick tree. पीलु *h. peeloo.*

(665) جبن JUBN. Cheese. *p. puneer.* پنير

(666) چنچرا CHIT-CHE-RA. चितचरा The inverted thorn. *p. khár-waz-gooneh.* خارواز کونه

(667) چچندا CHE-CHEEN-DÁ. चिचंडा A long kind of cucumber.

(668) جدوار JUD-WÁR. Zedoary. *vide* 398.

qu. hot and dry, 3. *prop.* an antidote against poisons. *ch.* China, which after grinding in water, is of a violet colour. *d.* half a direm to half a miskal. *cor.* coriander seed. *suc.* of zecumbád, three times the quantity.

(669) جدي JUD-EE. A kid. हलवान *h. hulwán. p. buz-gháleh.* بزغاله

(670) جرجيرالماء JIR-JER-UL-MÁA. A species of parsley, growing in marshy places.

(671) جراسيا JE-RÁ-SY-Á. Cherry. *p. áloo-bá-loo.* آلوبالو

(672) چراينا CHE-RÁY-TÁ. चरायता The wormseed plant. *a. kussub uz zereereh.* قصب الزريرة

(673) جرتوت JIRTOOT. The wild egg plant. *vide* 38 .

(674) جريث JEREES. The eel.

(675)

(675) جراد JE-RÁD. Locuft. ष्धिी h. *tiddee.* v. *mul-uck.* ملخ

qu. hot and dry, 2. *prop.* fudorific.

(676) جرادالبحر JE-RÁD-UL-BEHR. The fea locuft; a fhrimp. सिंगा h. *jheengá.* p. *mul-uck de-ree-á-iy.* ملخ دريابي

(677) جرجير JIRJEER. The herb rocket.

(678) جرجر JIR-JIR. A fpecies of bean. p. *ba-ké-lá.* باقلا

(679) چرونجي CHEROWNJEE. चरौनजी A fmall grain, refembling pepper. p. *nuckel khójeh.* نقل خواجه

(680) جزمازج JUZ-MÁ-ZUJ. Fruit of the tamrifk.

qu. hot and dry, 1.

(681) جزر JUZ-IR. Carrot. गाजर h. *gáj-ir.* p. *guz-ir.* كذر and *zirduck.* زردك

prop. deobftruent. *d.* 2 direms. *fuc.* turnips.

(682) جزربري JUZ-IR BIRREE, & JUZ-IR AKLEETEE. جزراقليتي Wild carrot. v. *fke-ká-kul.* شقاقل p. *zirduck defhtee.* زردكدشتي

(683) جست JUST जमन A fpecies of tin. p. *rouh tootyá.* روح توتيا

(684) جسمي JUSSMEE. A thorny plant. गुखरू h. *go-khroo.* v. *khár kuf-uck.* خارخسك

It bears a prickly fruit, of a triangular form.

(685) جعده JOA-DEH. A fpecies of wormfeed.

(686) چغندر CHOGHUNDER. *p.* Beet root. *a.* *fe-luck.* سلق

(687) جفتالبلوط JIST-UL-BE-LOOT. The outfide fkin of an acorn.

(688) جفري JEF-REE. The envelope of the bud of a female palm tree.

(689) جليد JE-LEED. Ice. घाला h. *pá-lá.* p. *berf.* برف

(690) جلد JILD. Skin, leather. चमरा h. *chumrá.* p. *poft.* پوست

prop. healing, and ftyptic. *ch.* the fkin of a fucking animal.

(691) جلنار JULNÁR. Flowers of the barren wild pomegranate tree.

qu. cold 1, dry 2. *prop.* aftringent. *h.* Perfian or Egyptian. *d.* 1 to 2 direms. *cor.* tragacanth, with oil of almonds.

(692) جلجلان JUL-JE-LAN. Dried coriander feed.

p. *kifh*

p. *kiſhnee khuſh.* كشنيزخشك

(6;3) جلنسرين JUL-NUS-REEN. The roſe of Jericho, or dogroſe.

p. *wurd-cheenee.* وردچيني

(694) جلنجبين JU-LEN GE-BEEN. Conſerve of roſes, made with honey.

p. *goolkund áſſulee.* كل قندعسلي

(695) چلغوزه CHILGHOZÁ. p. Pine kernels. चलगुजा h. *chil-go-já.*

(696) چلپاسه CHIL-PÁ-SEH. A Lizard. चिपकली h. *chip-kul-ee.*

(697) جلجلان الحبشي JULJULÁN-UL-HUBSHEE. Black poppy.

(698) جمست JUMUST. A kind of blue gem, found near Medina.

prop. cures palpitation of the heart, and fainting.

(699) جمد JUMED. a. Ice. *vide* 691. पाला h. *pá-lá.* p. *yekh.* يخ

(700) چهار JUMÁR. The pith of a palm tree. p. *puncer khurmá.* پنيرخرما

(701) جميز JUMEEZ. Adam's fig. *vide* 258. p. *injeer adam.* انجيرآدم

(702) جمل JUMEL. A camel. ऊंट h. *oonte* p. *ſhooter.* شتر

(703) جمسفرم JUM-US-FERIM. A ſpecies of ſweet baſil.

(704) جمان JUMÁN. A wood, the outſide of which is black, and the inſide of a piſtachio green. v. *jeeldaroo.* جيلدارو

prop. it deſtroys worms in the inteſtines.

(705) جمعيره JUM-EEREH. An Indian ſhrub. जहेंगरा h. *bhungrá.*

(706) جمدچيني JUM-ED CHE-NEE. Native alkaline ſalt. *vide* 129.

(707) جنطيانا JIN-TYÁ-NÁ. Gentian. *vide* 372.

qu. hot and dry 3. *prop.* deobſtruent, and diaphoretic. *ch.* Europe, of a reddiſh brown, and bitter taſte. *d.* half a miſkal. *cor.* ſpleenwort, or rhubarb.

(708) چنپا CHUMPÁ. चमपा An Indian flower tree.

prop. the ſeed is inebriating.

(709) جندبيدستر JUNDBEYDUS-TER. Caſtor.

p. *goond-bey-duſter.* كندبيدستر

qu. hot and dry 3. *prop.* attenuant, and diaphoretic. *d.* one quarter of a direm to one direm. *ſuc.* ſweet flag.

(710) چندن CHUNDUN. चंदन White ſandel wood.

p. *ſundul ſefeid.* صندل سفيد

(711) جوزبوا JOWZ BEWÁ Nutmeg. *vide* 660.

T

(712) جوزالطيب JOWZ UT TEIB.

The same as the above.

(713) جوزالمرج JOWZ UL MUR-
UJ. Winter cherry.

v. *hub kak-nej.* حب كاكنج

(714) جواكهار JEWÁ-KHÁR.

जवाखार Native alkaline falt

v. *nut-roon.* نطرون

(715) جوز JOWZ. Walnut. *vide* 46.

(716) چوك CHOOK. युक्त Sorrel.

p. *hum-áz.* حماض

(717) جوزماثل JOWZ MÁSSEL.

The thorn apple. धतूरा h. *dhé-toorá.*

p. *gooz gee-ah.* كوزكياه

> *qu.* cold and dry 4. *prop.* narcotic. *d.* one
> carat. *cor.* cotton.

(718) جوزالسرو JOWZ UL SIROE.

Fruit of the cyprefs tree.

> *qu.* hot and dry 3. *prop.* ftyptic. *d.* one
> direm to half a mifkal. *cor.* honey. *fuc.* pome-
> granate peels.

(719) جوانسا JEWN-WÁ-SÁ

जवांसा A thorny plant, of which
they make purdehs.

(720) جوزالكوثل JOWZ UL KOW
SUL.   The phyfic nut. मैनफल

h. *myn-phul.* p. *jowz ul kie.* جوزالغي

prop. emetic. *d.* one to two direms, in para-
lytic complaints. *fuc.* white hellebore.

(721) جوزالرت JOWZ-UL-RET.

A faponaceous nut. रीठा h. *ree.thá.*

(722) جوزهند JOWZ HIND. Cocoanut. नारयेल h. *nár-yel,* and खोपरा
kho-prá. p. *nárjeel.* نارجيل

(723) چولائي CHEW-LIE. चुलाई

An Indian pot-herb.

(724) چهر CHE-HUR. छड़ Spikenard.
vide 726.

(725) جهاوء J,HÁ-OU. झाउ Tamarifk tree. *vide* 36.

(726) چهتامانسي JEHTE-MÁN-
SEE. जटामासी Spikenard.

a. *fembel ut teib.* سنبل الطيب

(727) چينا CHEEN-TÁ. चीता

A red root, that is very acrid and
cauftic. p. *fhee-te-ruj.* شيطارج

(728) جيپال JY-PÁL. जैपाल

A purgative feed.

a. *hub-uf-ful-á-teen.* حب السلاطين

(729) جيلدارو JEEL-DÁ-ROO.

vide

(730) چيده CHEE-DEH. चीड़:

The leffer pine. a. *fenobir feghár.*

(731)

ح

(731) حاشا HÁSHÁ. Thyme.

(732) حاج HAJ. The thorny plant, from which is collected the fpecies of manna, called *terunjebeen: vide* 61:.

(733) حافر HÁFIR. Hoof of any animal. खुर h. *khur.* p. سم *foom. prop.* drying. *ch.* of clean animals. *cor.* oils. *fuc.* horn.

(734) حافظالنحل HAFIZ UL NEHUL. Euphorbium. *vide* 254.

(735) حب HUB. Berry, feed. बीज h. *beej.* फूल *phul.* p. دانه *daneh.* and *tokhem.* تخم

(736) حبحنكلا HUB HUNKILÁ. A grain refembling black pepper; but which withinfide is white and fweet. v. *hub fumneh.* حب السمنه

(737) حبةالسودا HUBBUT-UL-SOWDÁ. Black feed.
कलौंजी h. *kerownjee.* p. *fy-a da-neh.* سياه دانه

(738) حبةالخضرا HUBBUT-UL-KHUZRA. Fruit of the turpentine tree.

prop. diaphoretic, and provocative. *ch.* large, green, frefh.

(739) حبةالماء HUBEK-UL-MÁ. Water mint. p. *powdneh abee.* پودنه آبی

(740) حبالزبيب HUB-UZ-ZU-BEEB. Grape ftone.
दाख केबीज h. *dakh-key-beej.* p. *tokhem meveez.* تخم مويز

(741) حبالقلت HUB-UL-KILT. A fpecies of vetch. p. *mafh hindee.* कोलथी h. *kulthee.*

(742) حبةالتمساح HUBUK UL' TIMSÁH. Water mint; *vide* 739.

(743) حبالیهود HUB-UL-YE-HOOD. Winter cherry. *kahnuj.* كاكنج

(744) حبالعرعر HUB-UL UR-ÚR. Juniper berries.

(745) حبالصنوبرصغار HUB SENO-BIR SEGHAR. Fruit of the leffer pine. जोनद:केबीज h. *jundeh key beej.* p. *tokhem káj* تخم کاج and *ná-zow.* نازو

(746) حبالعصغر HUB UL USFER. Seed of fafflower.

(747)

(747) حب البقر HUBUCK-UL-BUCKIR. Camomile flowers. *vide* 235.

(748) حب الخروع HUB-UL-KHIR-WÁ. Seed of the palma christi.

ऊरंडेकेबीज h. *árundé key-beej.*

p. *tokhem beid injeer.* تخم بيد انجير

prop. discutient and emollient; and taken internally to carry off redundant humours, and for cleansing the blood. *d.* five to ten seeds, peeled.

(749) حبق HUB-UCK. Mint.

p. *powdeneh.* پودنه

(750) حب الملوك HUB UL MU-LOOK. A purgative seed.

p. *máhoodáneh.* ماهودانه

(751) حب النيل HUB-UL-NEIL. A purgative seed.

h. *tokhem kunkwá.* تخم كنكوا

(752) حب القلقل HUB-UL-KILKIL. Seed of wild pomegranate.

p. *tokhem ánár deshtee.* تخم انار دشتي

(753) حب الاثل HUB UL USSOL. Tamarisk berries. p. *guzmazuck* كزمازك

(754) حب السفرجل HUB US SU-FIRJUL. Quince seed.

बरीकेबीज h. *behee key beej.*

p. *beh-dá-neh.* بهدانه

qu. cold and moist. *ch.* of the four quince. *d.* two direms. *cor.* sugarcandy. *suc.* mallows seed.

(755) حب السلاطين HUB-US-SU-LÁTEEN. A purgative seed.

जमालगूट: h. *jemálgowtá.*

p. *doord.* دند

(756) حب البلسان HU-BUL BUL-SÁN. Carpobalsam.

p. *tokhem bulsán.* تخم بلسان

prop. attenuant, and cardiac; detergent. *d.* two direms.

(757) حب القطن HUB UL KOTEN. Cotton seed. बिनूला h. *beynowla.*

p. *pumbehdáneh.* پنبهدانه

(758) حب البان HUB-UL-BÁN. Ben nuts.

qu. hot and dry. *ch.* large, fragrant. *d.* two direms. *suc.* cassia lignea.

(759) حبه HUBBEH. A red seed, used as a weight by jewellers.

रत्ती h. *rutty.* p. *soorkh.* سرخ

(760) حب الراعي HUBBUCK-UR-RIEY. Mugwort. *vide* 73.

(761) حب سجستاني HUB SEJIS-TÁNEE. Cardamums.

(762) حب نبطي HUB-UCK NUB-TEE.

Garden mint.

p. *powdeneh boſtánee.* پودنهبستاني

(763) حبق صغري HUBUCK SUCK-REE, and حبق كرماني HUBUCK KERMÁNEE. Two names for ſweet baſil.

(764) حبق خراساني HUBUCK KHORASÁNEE. Sorrel.

(765) حجر اليشب HEJR UL YE-SHEB. Jaſper.

p. *ſung yeſhem.* سنك يشم

(766) حجر لابهت HEJR-UL-BE-HUT. The eagle ſtone. *vide* No. 242.

(767) حجر الافروج HEJR UL UF-ROOJ. Pumice ſtone.

(768) حجر اليهود HEJR UL YE-HOOD. Jew's ſtone, reſembling an olive. p. *ſung jehoodán.* سنك جهودان

(769) حجر البلور HEJR BELORE. Chryſtal. p. *ſung belore.* سنك بلور

(770) حجر البقر HEJR-UL-BUCK-IR. A ſtone found in the gall bladder of an ox. p. *gáwzereh.* كاوزهره

(771) حجر النسر HEJR UL NESR. The eagle ſtone. *vide* 242.

(772) حجر الدم HEJR UL DUM. Bloodſtone. v. *ſhádenej.* شادنج

(773) حجر القمر HEJR UL KUMR. The moon ſtone; *vide* 493.

चंदरकांत h. *chánderkánt.*

(774) حجر المغناطيس HEJR UL MICKNATEES. The loadſtone.

चोमुकपाहर h. *chumuck put hui*

p. *ſung ahun-no-bá.* سنك آهن ربا

qu. hot and dry. *ch.* of a dark red, and that attracts iron ſtrongly. *d.* half a miſkal to one direm.

(775) حجر الكرك HEJR UL KIRK. A white ſtone, found on the banks of the Indus.

(776) حجر الرخام HEJR UL RÚ-KAM. White marble.

(777) حجر الزيتون HEJR UL ZIE-TOON. The olive ſtone; another name for the Jew's ſtone. *vide* 768.

(778) حجر مشويه HEJR MESHEW-YEH. Lime. चुनाकली h. *chooná-kullee.* p. *nooreh.* نوره

(779) حجر قبطي HEJR KIBTEE. The Coptic ſtone; a kind of fuller's earth.

U

(780) حجرارمني HEJR URME-
NEE. Bole armenee.

v. *gil urmenee.* كل ارمني

prop. purgative. *d* half a direm to one mifkal.
cor. wafhing it.

(781) حجربحري HEJR BEH-REE.
Coral. *vide* 417.

(782) حدج HUD-UJ. Dried coloquintida. p. *hunzil khoofhk.* حنظل خشك

(783) حديد HE-DEED. Iron.

नोहा h. *lowha.* p. *á-bun.* آهن

(784) حراشارومي HIR-Á-SHÁ
ROOMEE. Wild muftard.

जंगलीराई h. *junglee rie.*

p. *khirdul bir-ee.* خردل رومي

(785) حرف الماء HERF-UL-MÁÁ.
A kind of water creffes.

(786) حرشف HIR-SHUF. Arti-
choke. v. *kungir.* كنكر

(787) حرف HERF. Seed of garden
creffes.

p. *tokhem turreh teyzuck.* تخم تره تيزك

(788) حرمل HERMUL. Seed of
wild rue. *vide* 114.

(789) حرجل HIRJUL. A fpecies of
locuft without wings.

(790) حسك HUS-UCK. A fmall
creeping plant.

qu. cold and dry, 1. *prop.* detergent, and deobftruent. *d.* two direms. *fuc.* fhepherd's ftaff.

(791) حشيش بزرالقطاونا HESHEESH
BUZIR-UL-KE-TOO-NA. Leaves
of fleawort. p. *birg bungoo.* برك بنكو

qu. cold and moift.

(792) حشيش الزجاج HESHEESH-
UZ-ZU-JAJ. A water plant.

p. *gee-ah áb-geenáh.* كياه ابكبينه

qu. cold and dry. *prop.* repellent. *d.* of the
juice ten direms.

(793) حشيش الطحال HESHEESH
UL TE-HÁL. Leaves of fpleenwort.
vide 141. p. *jungee dároo.* زنكي دارو

(794) حشيش خراساني HESHESH
KHORASANEE. Wormfeed.

p. *dermeneh khorafánee* درمنه خراساني

(795) حصرم HUSSRIM. Unripe
grapes. कच्चीदाख h. *kutchee dákh.*

p. *ghowrah ungeer.* غوره انكور

prop. aftringent. *cor.* anifeed and honey.
fuc. lemon juice.

(796) حضض HU-ZEEZ. Juice of lyi-
cum. रमवन h. *re-fowt.* p. *hu-lul.* هلل

prop. difcutient, fomewhat aftringent, and
ftyptic. *ch.* that of Mecca.

(797)

(797) حلبيب HULBEEB. A species of hermodactyls.

v. soorenjan hindee. سورنجان هندي

(798) حلتيت HILTEET. Asafœtida. vide 305.

(799) حلزون HULZOON. Conch shell. शंख h. sunkh. p. sunj. سنج

prop. drying.

(800) حلبه HULBEH. Fenugreek.

मेथी h. moohtee. v. shimlet. شبليت

qu. hot and dry. prop. suppurative, and emollient. d. two direms; and in clysters twenty direms. cor. oil of bitter gourd. suc. linseed.

(801) حماما HO-MÁ-MA. Amomum.

v. mahlooj. ماهلوج

prop. deobstruent, and detergent. ch. Armenian; of a bright yellow, and fragrant. d. two direms.

(802) حماض الارنب HUMAZ UL URNEB. Dodder. v. kushoos. كشوث

(803) حماض الاترج HUMAZ-UL-UT-REJ. Citron juice.

p. tursheh turenj. ترشه ترنج

qu. cold and dry. cor. poppy juice. suc. lemon juice.

(804) حماض البقر HUMAZ UL BUC-KIR. Wood sorrel. अम्लल

h. ámrool. p. humáz birree. حماض بري

(805) حماض نهري HUMÁZ NEH

REE. Garden sorrel. vide 813.

(806) حماض الامبر HUMZ-UL-A MEER. A small creeping plant.

(807) حمص HIM-IS. A kind of pulse.

चना h. che-na. p. nakhood. نخود

(808) حمض HIMIZ. a. Glasswort. vide 163.

(809 حمرالارض HUMR-UL' URZ. Earth-worm. p. kherateen. خراطين

(810) حمل HEML. A ram.

बकरा h. buckrá. p. bir-eh بره

(811) حمام HU-MAM. A pigeon.

परेवा h. purewá. p. kebooter. كبوتر

(812) حماض بستاني HUMÁZ BOS-TANEE. Garden sorrel. vide 806.

चुका h. chooká. p. toorsheenuck. ترشينك

(813) حمار اهلي HY-MÁR AHLEE. The common ass.

गदहा h. gud-há. p. khur خر

(814) حمار وحشي HYMAR WEH-SHEE. The onager, or wild ass.

p. gowr khur. كورخر

(815 حنا HINNÁ. The shrub cyprus, used in dying. मिनहदी h. minh dee.

prop.

prop. aftringent. d. for the cholic half a mifkal of the leaves; and as a cephalic two mifkals of the feed. cor. liquorice and tragacanth.

(816) حناي قريش HINNÁ-EY KO-REISH. Mofs that grows on ftones.

v huzáz us' fuckher. حزاز الصخر

(817) حنظل HUNZIL. Coloquintida.

vide 306. p. khirboozá telkh. خربزۀ تلخ

qu. hot 3, dry 2. prop. purgative, and deobftruent. ch. frefh, yellow, ripe. d. of the fruit from a carat to a direm; of the feed half a direm; or of the juice one dang and a half. cor. tragacanth, or maftich. fuc. wild rue.

(818) حنطه HINTEH. Wheat.

गेहूँ h. gee-hoon. p. gundum. کندم

(819) حندتوقي HUNDKOKEE. a. The fhrub lotus.

prop. attenuant, and diaphoretic. d. two direms. cor. endive.

(820) حوت HOOT. a. Fifh.

मछली h. mutchlee. v. a. fum-uck. p. máhee. ماهي سبک

(821) حواري HE-WA-REE. Wheat. flower. मैदा h. mydá. p. arud gundum. اردکندم

(822) حي العالم HY-UL-ÁLUM. Houfeleek.

(823) حيه HI-YEH. A fnake. सांप h. fámp, and नाग nág. p. már. مار

خ

(824) خامالانق الذيب KHÁ-MÁ-LA-UNECK'UZ-ZEEB. Wolf's bane.

(825) خانق الكلب KHÁNECK UL KELB. Dog's bane, a poifonous plant.

कुचला h. koo-che-lá. p. feloos máhee. فلوس ماهي

(826) خارپشت KHÁR-POOSHT. The porcupine. साही h. fy-hee. v. kunfuz. قنغذ

(827) خانق النمر KHÁNEK 'UN' NEMR. A poifonous plant: a fpecies of mezereon.

(828) خانق الملك KHÁNECK-UL-ME-LIC. Gall apple.

p. fá-dá-we-rán. ساداوران

(829) خاماءاقطي KHÁ-MÁ-ÁKTEE. Danewort.

(830) خبث الحديد KOOBS-UL-HE-DEED. Drofs of iron.

जो

लोदेकेकीट h. *lowhi key keet.* p. *reem áhun.* ریم آهن

(831) خبز KHUBZ Bread. *vide* 27.

(832) خبث النحاس KHOOBS-UL-NOHASS. Drofs of copper.

तांबेकेकीट h. *támbáh key keet.* p. *reem mifs.* ریم مسس

    qu. hot and dry 3. *prop.* aftringent, drying, cauftic.

(833) خبث الرصاص KHOOBS UL RESÁSS. Drofs of tin.

    p. *reem kullie.* ریم قلعي

    qu. cold and dry.

(834) خبث الغضه KHOOBS-UL-FIZ-EH. Drofs of filver.

    p. *cherk nokerá.* چرک نقره

(835) خبازي KHEBBAZEE. *a.* Mallows. *vide* 865.

(836) خرما KHURMÁ. Dates. *vide* 630.

(837) خربق اسود KHIRBUC US-WUD. Black hellebore.

कुतकी h. *kootkee.*

    qu. hot and dry 3. *prop.* purgative. *d.* half a direm. *cor.* oil of almonds, or tragacanth.

(838) خربق ابيض KHIRBUC ABI-YUZ. White hellebore.

p. *khirbuc fefeid.* خربت سفید

    qu. hot and dry 3. *prop.* emetic. *ch.* white, brittle, and pungent. *d.* half a direm. *cor.* maftich. *fuc.* nux vomica.

(839) خربوزه KHIRBOOZ. A grafs, ufed for dying yellow. p: *fupruc.* سبرک

(840) خروع KHIRWA. The palma chrifti plant. *vide* 84.

(841) خرفع KHIRFÁ. Fruit of the *Ág* tree. *vide* 248.

श्राककाफल h. *ág-ká-phul.*

(842) خرفق KHIRFUC. Seed of wild rue. *vide* 114.

(843) خرچنك KHIRCHUNG. *p.* Sea crab. केकरा h. *keynkerá.* p. *punj páiyeh.* پنج پایه

(844) خردل KHIRDUL. Muftard. राई h. *riey.*

    prop. heating, promoting digeftion, deobftruent.

(845) خراطين KHERÁ-TEEN. Earthworm. *vide* 276.

केंचुवा h. *keynchewá.*

    prop. promoting the growth of flefh in a wound.

(846) خراهين KHERU-HEEN. A leech. जोंक h. *joownk.* p. *zeloo.* ذلو

(847 خرفه KHURFA. Purflain. *vide* 433.

X

ले

लोनिआ h. *loonyá.*

(848) خرزهره KHIR-ZEREH. Rhododaphne.

(849) خرنوب‌شامي KHIRNOOB SHAMEE. A species of bean. Carobs.

qu. cold and dry. *prop* aftringent. *d.* five to ten direms. *fuc.* acorns.

(850) خرنوب‌نبطي KHIRNOOB NUBTEE. Carobs.

qu. cold and dry. *prop.* aftringent. *d.* 3 direms.

(851) خرنوب‌مصري KHIRNOOB MISREE. The fruit of the acorus thorn.

(852) خرنوب‌هندي KHIRNOOB HINDEE. Caffia fiftularis. *vide* 521.

(853) خردل‌فارسي KHIRDUL FARSEE. Seed of wild rue. *vide* 114.

(854) خس KHUSS. Lettuce.

p. *káboo.* كاهو

qu. cold and moift. *prop.* narcotic. *d.* two miſkals. *cor.* parfley. *fuc.* endive.

(855) خسرودارو KHUSROO-DA-ROO. Ganagal. *vide* 878.

(856) خسكدانه KHUSUC-DANEH. Seed of fafflower.

(857) خشكار KHOOSHKÁR. Un-sifted wheat flower. आटा h. *á-tá.*

(858) خشب‌الشونيز KHUSHUB-USH-SHOONEEZ. The black feed plant.

(859) خشخاش KHUSHKÁSH. Poppy. पोस्त h. *poft.* p. *kooknár.* كوكنار

(860) خصيةالثعلب KHUSYET-US'-SÁLEB. Satyrion.

qu. hot, and moift. *prop.* provocative. *d.* one to two miſkals. *cor.* myrobalans.

(861) خصيةالكلب KHUSYET-UL-KELB. A root refembling fatyrion.

(862) خصيةالبحر KHUSYET-UL-BEHR. Caftor. *vide* 164.

(863) خصيه KHUSYEH. Tefticle. पेजर h. *peyhlir.* p. *khá-yeh.* خايه

(864) خضلاف KHUZLÁF. The Bdellium tree.

p. *derukht mokul.* درخت‌مقل

(865) خطمي KHITMEE. Marfh mallows.

prop. emollient, and fuppurative. *eh.* that which bears a white flower. *fuc.* mallows.

(866) خغاش KHE-FÁSH. A bat. अमगीदर h. *chumgeedir.* p. *fhub-purrek.* شپرک

(867)

(867) خلد KHULID. A muſk rat.

चकचुनदरी h. *chuck-choondree.*

p. *mooſh khoor.* موش کور

(868) خلاق KHE-LAK. The willow.

p. *derukht beid.* درخت بید

qu. cold and dry. *prop.* drying *ch.* growing near a ſpring of water. *d.* of the juice twenty miſkals.

(869) خل KHULL. Vinegar.

p. *ſeerkeh.* سرکه

prop. attenuant. *cor.* ſugar, and oil of almonds.

(870) خلال KHELÁL. Unripe dates.

(871) خمر KHUMR. Grape wine.

ङाख्महद h. *dákh ká mudh.* p. *ſheráb*

ungooree. شراب انکوري

qu. hot and dry 3. *prop.* cordial. *d.* 72 miſkals.

(872) خمیر KHUM-EER. Leaven.

p. *khum-eer má-yeh.* خمیر مایه

(873) خمرالحمار KHUMR ' UL-HY-MÁR. A kind of ſoap aſhes.

साजी h. *ſajee.* p. *uſh-kár.* اشخار

(874) خمان KHÉ-MÁN. The elder tree.

(875) خذنی KHUNSÁ. Aſphodel.,

qu. cold and dry. *prop.* detergent. *d.* five direms of the leaves ; or of the buds and fruit two

direms. *ſuc.* valerian.

(876) خوخ KHOWKH. Peach.

p. *ſhooft-á-loo.* شغتالو

prop. correcting the bile.

(877) خوخ اقرع KHOWKH ÁK-RÁ.

Indian leaf. v. *ſádij hindee* سادج هندي

(878) خولنجان KHOW-LIN-JÁN.

Galangal. कोलीजन h. *koolinján.*

(879) خواجه کیاه KHOW JEH GEE-AH. An Indian ſhrub. बांसा h. *bán-ſá.*

(880) خیارشنبر KHY-A'R SHEM-BIR, and خیارچنبر KHY-A'R CHUMBIR. Caſſia fiſtularis.

अमलतास h. *amul-taſs.*

prop. purging bile. *ch.* Indian, black, full of grains, perfectly ripe, and with a thin ſkin. *d.* five to fifteen direms. *cor.* oil of almonds, and aniſeed, with an infuſion of tamarinds. *ſuc.* manna, with raiſins, and turbith root.

(881) خیار KHY-AR. Cucumber.

बीरा h. *kee-rá.*

p. *bád-rung.* باذرنک

qu. cold and moiſt.

(882) خیزران KYZ-RÁN. Rattan.

p. *choob beynt.* چوب بینت

qu. hot and dry. *prop.* expelling gravel *d.* two direms. *cor.* hempagrimony. *ſuc.* bramble root.

 د

(883) دارفلفل DÁR FILFIL. Long pepper. *vide* 18.

(884) دارشیشعان DÁR-SHEE-SHÁN. An acromatic bark. h. *ka-iy-phul.* कायफल

(885) داکه DÁKH. दाख Grapes. a. *in-ub.* عنب p. *ungoor.*

(886) دارچینی DÁR-CHEE-NEE. Cinnamon. दालचीनी h. *dal-cheenee.*

(887) دجاج DUJÁJ. The house hen. कुकरी h. *kuckree.* p. *má-keyán.* ماکیان

(888) دخن DOKHN. Millet. चीना h. *cheyná.* p. *arzun.* ارزن

(889) دخان DUKHÁN. Smoke. धूंआ h. *dhoon-án.* p. *dood.* دود

(890) دردی الخمر DOORDEE UL KHUMR. Dregs of wine. p. *doord sherab.* دردشراب

(891) درخت کلچکان DERUKHT GOOLCHUCKAN. The *mehwá* tree. महुवा h. *mehewá.*

(892) درمنه DIRMENEH. Worm-feed. *vide* 224.

(893) درونج عقربی DEROONUJ ÁK-RUBEE. A root, resembling the tail of a scorpion. अतुस h. *átus.* *qu.* hot and dry, 3. *prop.* attenuant, and cardiac. *d.* half to one direm. *cor.* aniseed. *suc.* civet.

(894) دستنبویه DUSTUMBOO-YEH. *p.* A small species of melon, very delicious. ककरी h. *cutchree.* a. *she-mám.* شمام

(895) دفلی DIFLEE. Rhododaphne. कनेर h. *ke-neir.* *qu.* hot and dry, 3. *prop.* discutient. *ch.* large leaves, very bitter. *d.* half a direm.

(896) دلب DOOLB. The plane tree. p. *derukht chenár.* درخت چنار *prop.* drying. *suc.* pomegranate peel.

(897) دم DUM. Blood. लहू h. *lohoo.* p. *khoon.* خون

(898) دماغ DE-MAGH. Brains. भिरेजा h. *bhey-ja.* p. *mughzsir.* مغزسر

(899) دم الاخوین DUM UL AKH-WEIN. Dragon's blood. बीर

हीरादुकी h. *heerá-dowkee.*

p. *khoon fy-owfhán.* خون سياوشان

prop. aftringent, and ftyptic. *d.* half a direm. *fuc.* gum arabic.

(900) دم الثعبان DUM US SO-BÁN. Another name for dragon's blood.

(901) دند DUND. A purgative feed. *vide* 387.

(902) دوسر DU-SIR. Wild wheat. *vide* 48.

(903) دود الحرير DOOD-UL-HER-EER. The filkworm. p. *ke-rem-ubreyfhum.* كرم ابريشم alfo *ke-rem-peelah.* كرم پيله

(904) دود القرمز DOOD UL KEER-MUZ. The *kermes* infect.

(905) دوض DOOZ. *a.* Water in which a red hot iron has been flaked.

(906) دوغ DOOGH. *p.* Buttermilk. छाच h. *ch,hátch,* and मठा *mut,há.*

(907) دوالك DEWÁLIK. A fpecies of mofs.

(908) دوم DOWM. The tree which yields bdellium.

p. *derukht mokul.* درخت مقل

qu. hot and dry. *prop.* fuppurative and attenuant. *eh.* frefh, of a yellow colour. *d.* one direm. *eor.* maftich.

(909) دونه تركي DOONEH TUR-KEE. A fpecies of anifeed.

जुरीअजवाई h. *jooree ájwein.*

(910) دهنيا D EHNYÁ. धनिया Coriander feed. p. *kifhneez.* كشنيز

(911) دهن DUHN. Oil. नेल h. *tail.* p. *roghen.* روغن

(912) ديك DEEK. The dunghill cock.

कुकर h. *ko-kir.* p. *kheroos.* خروس

(913) ديوك DEEWUCK. The white ant.

दीमक h. *deemuck.* a. *urzeh.* ارضه

(914) ديوچه DEWCHEH. *p.* The leech. जौंक h. *joownk.* p. *zéloo.* زالو

Y

ذ

(915) ذباب ZUBAB. The common fly. मखी h. *muck-hee.*
p. *mug-us.* مكس

qu. hot and dry. p. emollient and emetic.

(916) ذبل ZU-BUL. Tortoife-fhell.
p. *poft fungpoft.* سنك پشتـ

(917) ذراريح a. ZE-RA-REEH. Cantharides.

prop. bliftering. cor. new milk, and oil of almonds.

(918) ذلو ZE-LOO. The leech. *vide* 906.

(919) ذنب الغار ZENUB-UL FAR. Ribwort.

(920) ذهب ZEHUB. Gold.
सोना h. *fowna.* p. *zir.* زر

prop. cardiac. d. one carat of gold leaf. cor. honey and mufk.

(921) ذيب ZEEB. The wolf.
नेउरा h. *beruha.* p. *gurg* كرك

ر

(922) رانا RA-NA. a. Pomegranate.
रालेम h. *da-rim.* p. *anar.* انار a. *ruman.* رمان

(923) رازيانج RA-ZEE-A-NEJ. A fpecies of anifeed.

prop. deobftruent, and diaphoretic.

(924) راتينج رومي RA-TEE-NEJ ROOMEE. Turpentine of fir.
p. *zung-ba-ree.* زنكباري

(925) راوند RAWEND. Rhubarb.
रेवंचीनी h. *rey-wun cheence.* p. *rey-wend* ريوند

(929) راس RASS. The head of any animal.
मुनड h. *moond,* and *feer.* p. *fir.* سر

(927) رال RAL. Pitch. p. *keer.* قير

(928) راسن RA-SUN. Elecampane.

prop. attenuant. d. one mifkal.

(929) رب السوس RUB-US-SOOS. Liquorice juice.

v. *ufareh mehuc.* عصاره مهـك

(930) رشاد RE-SHAD. Garden creffes. हालिम h. *halim.*
p. *tur-eh teyzuc.* تره تيزك

(931)

(931) رصاص RE-SASS. Tin. *vide* 86.

(932) رطب RU-TUB. Dates.

p. *khurmá.* خرما

(933) رعي الجمام RA-IY UL HU-MÁM. Valerian.

(934) رقعه RUK-ÁH, Is the name of a red root; and in general it ufed to fignify all medicines that are applied to fractured limbs.

(935) ركت پهپ RUCKUT PHUP. रक्तफुप् The red-flowered Rho-dodaphne. लालकनेर h. *lálkeneer.* p. *khirzereh foorkh.* خرزهره سرخ

(936) رماد RE-MÁD. Afhes. राख h. *rákh.* p. *khá-kifter.* خاكستر

prop. drying. *ch.* the afhes of acorns. *d.* half a direm.

(937) رمان البر RUMÁN UL BIR. A tree refembling the pomegranate, but fmaller. The feed is called *hub kilkel.* The root thereof is called *mughar.*

(938) رمان حامض RUMÁN HUMÁZ. The four pomegranate. p. *anár toorfh.* انارترش

qu. cold and dry. *d.* ten wuckyeh of the juice. *fuc.* juice of unripe grapes.

(939) رند RUND. The laurel. *v.* *mowrid.* مورد

(940) رنف RUNF. An odoriferous plant. *v. beid mifhk.* بيدمشك

(941) روپا RU-PA. रुपा Silver. p. *nok-rá.* نقره

(942) روناس RU-NÁS. Madder. मजीठ h. *mé-jeeth.*

(943) روباه تربك RO-BÁ TUR-BUC. Nightfhade. *v. inub us fá-leb.* عنب الثعلب

(944) روي ROW-EY. A kind of brafs. कांसा h. *kán-fá.* a. *foofr.* صفر

(945) رهشي REH-SHEE. Sefamé meal.

(946) ریباس REE-BASS. The rhu-barb root, or rhapontic.

(947) ريش REESH. A feather. पंख: h. *punkh.* p. *pur.* پر

(948) ريحان RI-HAN. Sweet bafil. काली तुलसी h. *ká-lee tulfee.* p. *naz-bu.* نازبو

(949) ريه REE-YEH. The lungs. फेफरा h. *phephrá.* p. *fhufh.* شش

(950)

ز

(950) زاج ZAJ. General name for all the kinds of vitriol.

(951) زبيب ZE-BEEB. Raisins. किशमिश h. *kishmish.* p. *me-weez.* مويز

prop. emollient, and suppurative. *d.* ten direms. *suc.* jujules.

(952) زبد ZUBD. Butter. मरवन h. *muckhun.* p. *muskeh.* مسکه

(953) زباد ZUBÁD. Civet.

(954) زبدالبحر ZUBD'UL-BEHR. Foam of the sea. समंद्रफेन h. *semunder-pheen.* p. *kefdery-á.* کفدریا

prop. detergent. *ch.* yellow. *d.* one to two dangs. *suc.* bole armenic.

(955) زبل ZIBL. Dung. लीद h. *leed.* p. *sirgeen.* سرکین

(956) زجاج ZUJAJ. Glass. *vide* 26.

(957) زدوار JUDWÁR. Zedoary. v. *judwár.* جدوار

(958) زراوندمدحرج ZERAWEND MUDEHRUJ. Round birthwort. p. *zerawund geerd.* زراوندکرد

prop. attenuant, and deobstruent. *ch.* thick, of a saffron colour. *d.* one miskal to two direms. *cor.* honey. *suc.* zerumbád.

(959) زراوندطويل ZERA-WEND TE-WEEL. Long birthwort. p. *zerawend dráz.* زراونددراز

prop. deobstruent, discutient, and healing. *ch.* of a saffron colour, and thicker than the thumb.

(960) زرنيخسرخ ZER-NEEKH SOORKH. Red orpiment. *vide* 113.

(961) زرنباد ZERUMBAD. कचूर h. *kutchoor.*

prop. attenuant, cardiac, and tonic. *d.* one direm.

(962) زرنيخزرد ZER-NEEKH ZIRD. Yellow orpiment. *vide* 101.

prop. corrosive; poisonous.

(963) زرسود ZIR-SOOD. Turmeric. हलदी h. *huldee.* p. *zird choobeh.* زردچوبه

(964) زرير ZIREER. Milelot. *vide* 138.

(965) زرشك ZERISHK, and ZE-RUNG. زرنك Barberries.

(966) زرتك ZIR-TUCK. Juice of safflower. रंगकुसंभ h. *rung-kesumbh.* p. *áb khufac.* آبخسق

(967) زعرور ZU-ROOR. The medlar. p. *ke-yul.* کيل

prop. astringent. *ch.* red, ripe.

(968) زعفران ZÁ-FRÁN. Saffron.

कि

केसर   h. *key-fir.*

prop. difcutient, deobftruent, fuppurative, ex-hilirating, and narcotic.   *d* half to one direm. *cor.* anifeed.

(969) زغال ZU-GHAL. Charcoal. कोइला h. *koeyla.*

(970) زغن ZUGHUN. The kite. चील h. *cheel.* p. *gluleewa'z.* غليواز

(971) زفت ZIFT. Pitch.

prop. difcutient and detergent. *ch.* clean and gloffy. *fuc.* epoponax.

(972) زقوم ZÉ-KOOM. A thorny tree. सिहंद h. *fynhud,* and थोर *thew-er.*

(973) زمرد ZUM-U-RUD. Eme-rald. पन्ना h. *punna.*

(974) زنجبيل رطب ZUNJEBEEL RUTB. Green ginger *vide* 55.

(975) زنجار ZUNJÁR. Verdegris. p. *zungár.* زنكار

prop. detergent.

(976) زنجفر ZUNJEFIR. Cinnabar. ईंगुर *ingoor.* p. *fhungerf.* شنكرف

prop. poifonous. *cor.* ghee and warm water.

(977) زنكبار ZUNGBÁR. Blue vitriol. नीलाथोथा h. *nee-la tho-tha'.*

(978) زنجرف ZUNJERF. Cinna-bar. *vide*

(979) زنجبيل ZUNJEBEEL. Dry ginger. सोंठ h. *fownth.*

(980) زنكار معدني ZUNGAR MAADENEE. Green vitriol. p. *tootya fubz.* توتياي سبز

(981) زنجبيل شامي ZUNJEBEEL SHAMEE. Elecampane. v. *rá-fun.* راسن

(982) زوفاء رطب ZU-FÁ-IY RUTB.

A filthy fubftance found on the tails of the Armenian fheep, faid to be ow-ing to their feeding on a milky kind of grafs, that is very heating.

prop. fuppurative, and emollient. *ch.* very greafy. *cor.* rofes.

(983) زوفاي يابس ZU-FA-IY YE-A-BUS. Hyffop.

prop. attenuant, fuppurative, diaphoretic, and deftroying worms in the inteftines. *ch.* that which is brought from Jerufalem. *cor.* gum ara-bic. *fuc.* mint and maiden hair.

(984) زيرا ZEE-RA. जीरा Cu-min feed. a. *ki-moon.* كمون

Z   (985)

(985) زیت ZI-ET. Olive oil.

ch. fresh. *cor.* honey.

(986) زیبق ZEE-BUC. Quickfilver. *vide* 15.

qu. hot and dry. *prop.* hurtful. *ch.* that which has never been ufed.

(987) زیتون ZIE-TOON. The olive tree and fruit. जलपाई *h. julpaiy.*

س

(988) ساج SÁJ. A foreft tree. साल *h. fál.*

(989) سابر SA-BIR. साबर An Indian animal, whofe fkin is ufed for fword fcabbards.

(990) ساذج هندي SÁDIJ HIN-DEE. Indian leaf. तेजपात *h. teyj-pát.*

(991) سارس SÁ-RESS. An Indian bird, of the ftork kind. सारस

(992) سانبهرلون SÁMBHER-LOON. सांबरनोन Rock falt.

(993) ساکون SÁ-GOON. सागुन An Indian tree, whofe leaves are compared to elephant's ears.

(994) ساجي SÁ-JEE. साजी A kind of foap afhes.

(995) ساتهي SÁTHEE. साटी A fpecies of red rice.

(996) سبح SUB-EH. Jet.

p. fheb-eh. شبه

(997) سپستان SEEPISTÁN. Sebeftens. लसोरा *h. lehfoorá.* *p. fugpiftán.* سكپستان

prop. emollient and fuppurative. *ch.* full of pulp. *d.* 16 to 30. *cor.* myrobalans. *fuc.* jujubes.

(998) سپندان SE-PEN-DÁN. Wild rue. *vide* 114.

(999) سپاري SU-PÁ-REE. सुपारी Areca nut; betelnut. *a. fonful.* فوفل

(1000) سداب SUD-ÁB. Rue. सातरी *h. fá-tu-ree.*

prop. difcutient, diaphoretic, and anthelmentic. *d.* three direms. *cor.* anifeed.

(1001) سدر SEYDIR. A fpecies of plum tree. बेरकारूख *h. beyr ka'rookh.* *p. derukht konár.* درخت کنار

prop. aftringent. *ch.* broad leaves. *d.* three direms of the leaves. *cor.* tragacanth.

(1002) سرب SOORB. Lead. सीसा *feefá.*

(1003)

(1003) سرنج SOO-RUNJ. Red lead.
vide 120.

(1004) سرخس SIRUKHS. A black root.

prop. deobftruent, and drying. *ch.* black, and large, with the infide of a piftachio green.

(1005) سرشف SIR SHUF. Muftard.

सरसून *h. fir-foon.*

(1006) سرمق SIR-MUC. Orach.
vide 403.

(1007) سرو SIR-OE. The cyprefs tree.

(1008) سرطان SIRTAN. The crab. *vide*

ch. the water crab.

(1009) سركه هندي SIR-KEH HIN-DEE. Bread foaked in water, and kept in the fun till it becomes four.
vide 25.

(1010) سعد SOAD. Root of an odoriferous grafs. मोथा *h. mowt,ha.*

prop. diaphoretic, cardiac and tonic. *ch.* that brought from Cufah. *d.* one direm. *fuc.* cinnamon and fweet flag.

(1011) سعتر SA-TUR. An odoriferous plant. साहर *h. fit,her.*

(1012) سفرجل SUFIR-JUL. Quince.
vide 28.

prop. aftringent, ftyptic, cardiac, and tonic. *d.* ten direms of the juice. *cor.* dates, or honey. *fuc.* pears.

(1013) سقمونیا SUC-MOO-NYA. Scammony.

मह मूद *h. meh-moo-deh.*

prop. cathartic. *ch.* that brought from Antioch; clean and light, gloffy, of the colour of raw-filk, and eafily friable. *d.* a carat, to two dangs.

(1014) سكبینج SUG-BEE-NUJ. Gum fagapenum.

prop. deobftruent, attenuant, and expelling gravel and ftone. *d.* one direm to one mifkal. *cor.* liquorice.

(1015) سكر SUKHIR. Sugar.

चीनी *h. chenee.* *p. fhuckir.* شكر

prop. detergent, and emollient. *d.* twenty direms.

(1016) سكانكور SUG UNGOOR. Dog's grapes; nigthfhade.

a. inub us faleb. عنب الثعلب

(1017) سكنجبین SE-KUN-JE-BEEN. Oxymel of vinegar and honey.

prop. emetic.

(1018) سلت الماء SULK-UL-MAA. A water plant. *vide*

(1019) سلت SELT. A fpecies of barley. *p. jow bir,he,neh.* جوبرهنه

(1020) سلاجت SA-LA-GET. A fpecies of ftorax.

(1021) سلاریس SIL-ARRUS. Liquid

ftorax

ftorax. v. *me-áy-fá-ye-leh.* میعهسایله

(1022) سلق SULK. Beet root.

p. *chogbundir.* چغندر

> *prp.* difcutient, attenuant, .detergent. *ch.* white. *cor.* vinegar. *f,c.* turners.

(1023) سلم SUL-UM. The gum arabic tree. *vide* 400.

(1024) سلجمي SULJUM. Turnep. p. *fhul-ghum.* شلغم

> *prp.* diaphoretic. *fuc.* carrots.

(1025) سلیخه SE-LEE-KHEH. Caf-fia lignea. तज h. *tuj.*

(1026) سم SUM. Poifon in general. बिस h. *bifs.* p. *ze-her.* زهر

(1027) سم الحمار SUM-UL-HYMÁR. Rhododaphne.

(1028) سم الغار SUM-UL-FÁR. Rat's bane. Realgar.

p. *murgh moofh.* مرکموش

(1029) سمور SUN-OOR. The fable, or marten. *vide* 332.

(1030) سمندر SEMUNDER. The falamander.

(1031) سباروغ SE-MA-ROUGH. Mufhroom.

(1032) سماق SU-MÁK. Sumach.

> *prep.* aftringent, and cardiac. *ch.* frefh, and red. *cor.* maftich. *fuc.* lemon juice.

(1033) سماق SE-MÁK. A fmall grain. कंगनी h. *kungnee.*

(1034) سمک SE-MUC. Fifh. मछली h. *mutchlee,* and मीन *meen.* p. *má·hee.* ماهي

(1035) سم السمک SUM-UL-SE-MUC. A poifonous milky grafs, bearing a yellow flower.

p. *má-hee ze-ruj.* ماهي زیرج

(1036) سمسم SOM-SOM. Sefamê feed. तिल h. *til.* p. *kunjed* کنجد

(1037) سمن SE-MUN. Ghee. घी h. *ge-hew.* p. *roghen gáw.* روغنگاو

(1038) سمن SU-MUN. The lily of the valley.

(1039) سمندرلون SEMUNDER-LOON. समुद्रलोन Sea falt.

p. *nemuc de-ry-á.* نمکدریا

(1040) سنا SUN-A. Senna.

> *p.* cathartic. *ch.* that which grows about Mecca. *d.* 4 to 7 direms in infufion, or in fubftance 3 direms. *cor.* yellow myrobalans, rofe leaves, gum arabic, and tragacanth.

(1041)

(1041) سنكهارا SIN.GHA.RÁ. सिंघारा
A prickly fruit.

It is of a triangular form, about the size of a filbert, and is produced by a plant that grows on the surface of the water.

(1042) سنبل الطيب SEMBEL UT-TIEB. Indian spikenard.

(1043) سنجاب SON-JÁB. The grey squirrel.

(1044) سنور SE-NORE. The cat. बिल्ली h. billee. p. goorbeh. کربه

(1045) سندروس SUNDROOS. Sandarach.

prop. drying. ch. transparent. d. half a miskal.

(1046) سن SUN. सन Hemp. a. kennub. قنب

(1047) سنكه SUNKH. संख Conch shell. p. sefeid mohreh. سفیدمهره

(1048) سنبل هندي SEMBEL HIN-DEE. Indian spikenard. vide 1042.

(1049) سنبل رومي SEMBEL ROO-MEE. Celtic nard. v. nardeen. ناردين

(1050) سوسپند SOOSPUND. A species of milky grass. दोदिही h. dood-hee. p. sheer-geeáh. شیرکیاه

(1051) سوسمار SOOSMAR. The guana. गुदासाँफ h. go-eh samph.

(1052) سویق SÁ-WECK. Any grain fried and then ground into flour. सातू h. sá-too.

(1053) سورنجان SU-REN-JÁN, Hermodactyls. vide 179.
जंगलीसिंघारा h. junglee singhárá.

(1054) سوسن SO-SUN. The lily.

(1055) سونچرلون SOWNCHUR-LOON. सोंचलोन Salt of bitumen. p. nim-uck see-áh. نمکسیاه

(1056) سورن SOORUN. सोरं An Indian root, called also BUJ-IR-KUND. बज्रकंद

(1057) سونته SOWNT.H. सोंठ Dry ginger. p. zunjebeel. زنجبیل

(1058) سوري SOOREE. सोरी A species of red vitriol, used by shoemakers.

(1059) سهاگا SO-HÁ-GÁ. सुहागा Tincal. p. tin-kár. تنکار

(1060) سهورا SEHOWRÁ. सहोरा An Indian tree, which it is pretended

A a

no fnake will approach.

(1061) سير SEER. Garlic.

लहसुन h. *lehfun.*

(1062) سيكران SIEK-RÁN. Black henbane feed. a. *buzir-ul-bung.* بزرالنج

(1063) سيندهالون SINDAHLOON.

मेंदा लोनू Rock falt. p. *nimuck fung.* نمكسنك

(1064) سيسون SEE-SOON. सिसुन An Indian foreft tree.

(1065) سياهدانه SEE-AH DÁNEH. Black feed. कलौंजी h. *kelownjee.*

ش

(1066) شاهلوج SHAHLOOJ. A fpecies of yellow plum. p. *fhah áloo.* شاه آلو

(1067) شاهترج SHÁHTERUJ. Fumitory. पित्पापरा h. *pit-páp-rá.* p. *fháhtereh.* شاهتره

    prop. deobftruent, detergent, and cathartic. *ch.* green, bitter. *d.* of the juice half a rutel. *cor.* lemon juice and honey. *fuc.* ½ the weight of fenna.

(1068) شاماخ SHAMÁKH. A grain. सांवां h. *fan-wa.*

(1069) شاهانجير SHAHINJEER. A fpecies of fig. p. *injeer vizeeree.* انجيروزيري

(1070) شاهبلوط SHÁH BELOOT. Acorns. v. *beloot ul melic* بلوطالملك

    prop. aftringent. *cor.* fugar, or honey. *d.* two direms.

(1071) شاهدانق SHÁHDÁNUC. The inebriating hemp feed. p. *tokhem bung.* تخم بنك

(1072) شادنج SHADENUJ. Bloodftone.

(1073) شالوك SHÁHLOOK. शालुक An Indian root.

(1074) شاهسغرم SHÁ-HUS-FÉ-RUM. Sweet bafil. v. *ri-hán.* ريحان

(1075) شاهبوي SHAH-BOO. Ambergris. v. *umbir.* عنبر

(1076) شانهدشتى SHÁ-NEH DESHTY. The comb tree, *vide* 590. कंगसी h. *kung h-nee.*

(1077) شب SHUBB. Alum. *vide* 575.

(1078) شبت SHIB-IT. Fennel. सोवा h. *fow-á.*

    prop. fuppurative, and narcotic. *d.* two direms.

(1079) شبرم SHIB-REM. A fpecies of fpurge.

(1080)

(1080) شبيبي SHE-BI-BEE. A narcotic root. The inebriating hemp-seed also bears this name.

(1081) شجرةالدب SHEJERUT'UL-DUB. The bear's tree; the medlar tree.

(1082) شجرةالحبات SHEJERUT ULHY-ÁT. The tree of life; the cypress.

(1083) شجرةالبراغيث SHEJERUT UL BERÁGHEES. Hemp agrimony.

(1084) شجرةالموسي SHEJERUT UL MOOSA. Moses's bush; the bramble.

(1085) شحم SHE-HUM. Grease of any animal.

चर्बी h. chirbee. p. peeh. پيه

(1086) شحمحنظل SHE-HUM HUN-ZEL. The pulp of the coloquintida fruit. p. mughz hunzel. مغزحنظل

prop. emollient.

(1087) شراب SHÉ-RÁB. p. Wine; also all kinds of sherbets.

(1088) ششترة SHESHTEREH. Valerian. v. fooh. فوه

(1089) شعير SHE-EER. Barley.

p. jow. جو

(1090) شعر SHÁIR. Hair.

बाल h. bál.　　　p. moo. موي

(1091) شتاقل SHE-KÁ-KUL. Wild carrot.

(1092) شقايقالنعمان SHE-KA-YEK-UL-NÁMÁN. The anemone.

p. gool lá-leh. كل لاله

(1093) شلجم SHULJUM. Turnep.

p. shulghum. شلغم

(1094) شبليت SHIM-LEET. Fenugreek. मेथी h. meet hee.

(1095) شمشاد SHUMSHÁD. The box tree.

(1096) شمع SHUMÁ. Bees wax.

p. moom. موم h. mehdoomul. मघुमैन

(1097) شنبليد SHUMBELEED. Flower of the hermodactyl plant.

p. gool soorenján. كل سورنجان

(1098) شونيز SHOONEEZ. Black-seed. p. see-ah dáneh. سياهدانه

prop. detergent, destroying worms, discutient, and diaphoretic. d. half a miskal to two direms.

(1099) شوكران SHOWKERÁN. Black henbane seed.

p. tokhem bung roomee. تخم بنكارومي

(1100)

(1100) شوكه SHOWKH. A thiftle.
ऊंटकेतारा h. *oont-ké-tá-rá*.

(1101) شيرخشت SHEERKISHT. A fpecies of manna, which is collected from a barren tree called *derukt bey cheub*, growing in Khorafan.

prop. cathartic. *ch.* tranfparent, like gum arabic. *d* 7 to 30 direms.

(1102) شيطرج SHEE-TERUJ. An Indian plant.
श्रीन: h. *cheeth*. p. *fhee-tureh* شيتره

prop. detergent. *ch.* Indian. *d.* one mifkal. *cor.* maftich. *fuc.* valerian.

(1103) شيح SHEEH. Wormfeed.

p. *dirmeneh*. درمنه

prop. deftroying worms, and deobftruent. *ch.* Armenian. *d.* half a direm. *fuc.* wormwood.

(1104) شيربخشير SHEER-BUCK-SHEER. A yellow root growing in Hindoftan and Cafhmeer.
हरबी h. *hirbee*.

(1105) شبرخشك SHEER-KHOOSHK. A fpecies of manna collected from the willow in Khorafan.
p. *beid khifht.* بيدخشت and *beid angee-been.* بيدانكبيين

(1106) شيلم SHYLUM. Tares.

ص

(1107) صابون القاف SÁBOON-UL-KÁF. Soap afhes.
v. *chowbuck ufhnán* چوبك اشنان

(1108) صابون SÁ-BOON. Soap.

prop. cauftic, and detergent. *ch.* old. *fuc.* lime and foap afhes.

(1109) صبر SYB-IR. Aloes. *vide* 344.

prop. drying; caufing flefh to grow; cathartic. *ch.* focoterine. *d.* to thirty direms. *cor.* gum arabic, and tragacanth.

(1110) صداءالحديد SUDEED-UL-HEDEED. Iron ruft.
p. *záfrán áhun.* زعفران آهن

(1111) صدف SUD-UF. Any fhell.
सीपी h. *fee-pee.*

prop. drying. *d.* one mifkal, or of lime-water three direms. *cor.* honey and jujubes.

(1112) صدپيوند SUD-PY-WUND. Shepherd's ftaff.
v. *ufhur ur rá-iy.* عصرالراعي

(1113) صعتر SÁ-TUR. Origanum.

p.

p. *ouſhneh.* اوشه

(1114) صل SEL. The adder. A ſnake that will not be enchanted.

(1115) صمغ SUMEGH. Gum in general. गोंद h. *goondh.*

    prp. aſtringent. *ch.* gum arabic.

(1116) صمغ السداب SUMEGH U'S SUDÁB. Gum of rue.

(1117) صمغ الحروث SUMEGH-UL-MEHROOS. Aſafœtida.

v. hilteet. حلتيت *vide* 305.

(1118) صمغ القثاد SUMEGH UL KUSSÁD. Tragacanth. *v. keſeeerá* كثيرا

(1119) صمغ عربي SEMUGH ÁRE-BEE. Gum arabic. *vide* 1115.

(1120) صندل احمر SUNDUL AH-MER. Red Sandel wood.

रक्तचंदन h. *ruckut chundun.*

p. *ſundul ſoorkh.* صندل سرخ

(1121) صنوبر كبار SENOBIR KO-BÁR. The large pine.

p. *derukht chulghozeh.* درخت چلغوزه

    prop. fattening. *ch.* freſh, large, white. *d.* fifteen kernels.

(1122) صنوبر صغار SE-NO-BIR SEGHÁR. The leſſer pine.

(1123) صندل ابيض SUNDUL ABI-YUZ. White ſandel wood.

चंदन h. *chundun.*

p. *ſundul ſefeid* صندل سفيد

    prop. cordial. *d.* half a miſkal.

(1124) صوف SOOF. Wool. ऊन h. *oon.* p. *puſhm.* پشم

(1125) صوطله SOO'TLEH. A ſpecies of beet.

ض
—

(1126) ضان ZÁN. A ſheep. नेड़ h. *bheir.*   p. *meiſh* ميش

(1127) ضفدع ZUFDEH. A frog. मेंडूक h. *meidook.*   p. *ghowk.* غوک

B b

(1128)

طا & ظا

(1128) طاوُس TÁOUS. A peacock. मोर h. *moor.*

(1129) طبرزد TUB-IR-ZUD. Sugar candy.

(1130) طباشِير TE-BÁ-SHEER. Sugar of bamboo. *vide* 546.

   prop. drying, cardiac and tonic. *d.* two dangs in rofe water. *fuc.* half the weight of camphor.

(1131) طحلب TOHLUB. Water mofs.

   prop. repellent. *ch.* what grows on fweet water.

(1132) طرفا TURFÁ. The tamarifk tree. *vide* 36.

   prop. aftringent, and drying. *ch.* that which grows at fome diftance from water. *d.* five direms. *cor.* oil of almonds and honey.

(1133) طراثيث TERASEE'S. *a.* Name of a fruit. *p. bil.* بل

   prop. aftringent. *ch.* white. *d.* two mifkals. *cor.* tragacanth.

(1134) طرثوث TURSOOS. A thorny tree which produces the gum ammoniac. *p. derakht ufhuc.* درخت اشق

(1135) طرخون TURKHOON. *a.*

Tarregon, or dranculus hortenfis. *vide* 1210.

(1136) طلا TE-LÁ. Gold; alfo old wine. *vide* 596.

(1137) طلق TULK. Talc. अबरक h. *ubhruc.* *a. kokub ul urz.* كوكب الارض

   prop. aftringent. *cor.* oil and warm water.

(1138) طهف TEHF. A grain. *v. zoorut.* ذرت

(1139) طين احمر TEEN AHMER. Red earth.

गेरू h. *geeroo.* *p. gil foorkh.* كل سرخ

(1140) طين شاموش TEEN SHÁ MOOSH. Samian earth.

(1141) طين مختوم TEEN MUKHTOOM. Sealed earth.

   prop. aftringent, and cordial. *d.* two direms.

(1142) طين TEEN. Earth; bole. मट्टी h. *mittee.* *p. gil.* كل

(1143) طين ارمني TEEN URMENEE. Bole armenic.

p. gil urmenee. كل ارمني

(1144) طين‌قبرسي TEEN KUB-RUSSEE. Cyprus earth.

(1145) طين‌فارسي TEEN FARSEE. Persian earth, ufed for cleanfing the head. p. *gil firfhew.* كل‌سرشوي

(1146) ظبي ZUBBEE. A deer. हिरन h. *hurn.* p. *áhoo.* آهو

(1147) ظفيره ZU-FEERÁH. Wild mint.

p. *powdeneh birree.* پودنه‌بري

(1148) ظلف ZILF. The hoof of any animal.

खूर h. *khoor.* p. *foom.* سم

(1149) ظيان ZY-ÁN. Wild jafmin: जाहीजूई *jáhee-jewhee.* p. *yáfmeen birree.* ياسمين‌بري

prop. cauftic. *or.* oil of rofes. *fuc.* laurel and fquills.

ع

(1150) عاقرقرحا AKIR-KER-HÁ. Dranculus.

prop. difcutient, and attenuant. *eb.* pungent. *d.* two dangs. *cor.* raifins, or liquorice.

(1151) عاج AWJ. Ivory. हाथी‌दान्त h. *hát hee dánt.* p. *den-dán feel.* دندان‌فيل

prop. drying. *d.* half a direm rafped.

(1152) عبهر UBHIR. The narciffus. p. *nurgis.* نرگس

(1153) عبير A-BEER. Saffron. v. *fafran.* زعفران

(1154) عتم UT-UM. The wild olive. p. *zietoon kouhee.* زيتون‌كوهي

(1155) عدس‌مر UD-US MURR. The bitter pea. p. *mufheng telkh.* مشنك‌تلخ

(1156) عرطنيثا UR-TÁ-NEE-SÁ. Sowbread. *vide* 407, and 543.

(1157) عروق‌حمرا U-ROOK-HUMRÁ. Madder.

(1158) عرطب URTUB. A fmall creeping plant. *vide* 790. p. *huffuck.* حسك

(1159) عرعر UR-UR. The mountain pine.

(1160) عروق‌الصفر U ROOK-US-SEFR. Turmeric. *vide* 1153.

prp.

prop. difcutient, attenuant, and diaphoretic.
ch. hard.   *d.* half a direm.

(1161) عروق U-RCOK. Roots in general. p. *beiykh-ha.* بیخہا

(1162) عروسک É-RCO-SUC. A fmall infect, of a beautiful fcarlet colour. बिरबोटी   h. *beer-be-howtee.*

(1163) عروق الصباغین U-ROOK US SE-BÁGHEEN. Turmeric. p. *zirdchowbeh.* زردچوبہ

(1164) عروسک دربردہ UR-OO-SUC-DIR-PIRDEH. Winter cherry. *vide* 443.

(1165) عزیز UZ-EEZ. Centaury.

(1166) عسل القصب USSUL UL KUSSEB. Juice of the fugar cane. रस h. *rufs.*   p. *fheereh nei fhuckir.* شیرہ نیشکر

(1167) عسل النحل USSUL-UL-NEHL. Honey. मधु h. *mudhoo.*   p. *fhehud.* شہد
prop. detergent, and heating.   *ch.* of a light yellow, pure, and fragrant.

(1168) عصارہ USSA-REH. Expreff-ed juice. p. *ufshoordeh.* افشردہ

(1169) عصفر USFIR. Safflower. *vide* 44.

(1170) عصفور US-FOOR. A Sparrow. p. *kunjufhk.* کنجشک

(1171) عصی الراعی UESÚR-RAIY. Shepherd's ftaff.   *vide* 61.

(1172) عضاة UZ-UT. General name for thorny plants.

(1173) عضرس IZRISS. Wild mal-lows.   p. *khitmee birree.* خطمی بری

(1174) عضل UZUL. The field moufe.   p. *mofh-kuc.* مشکک

(1175) عظم UZM. Bone. हड्डी h. *huddee.* p. *uftukhán.* استخوان

(1176) عظلم IZLUM. The Indigo plant.   p *derukht neel.* درختنیل

(1177) عفص ÚF-ES. Gall apple. माजूफल h. *májoophul.* p. *mazoo.* مازو
prop. aftringent and ftyptic.   *ch.* green, not per-forated.   *d.* half a direm.

(1178) عقرب UKRUB. A fcorpion. बिछू h. *beechew.* p. *khezjhem.* کزدم
prop. expelling gravel.

(1179) عقیق UKEEK. A cornelian.
prop. drying.   *ch.* thofe found in Yemen, that

are

are very red and tranſparent. *d.* half a direm. *ſuc.* amber.

(1180) علث ILSS. Wild ſuccory. p. *káſ-nee birree.* كاسني بري

(1181) عليق U-LIEK. The bramble. p. *toot-ſeh gúl.* توتسه کل

    prop. aſtringent. *d.* of the root three direms. *cor.* liquorice root. *ſuc.* pomegranate buds.

(1182) علك بغدادي UL-UK BÁGHDÁ-DEE. Maſtich.

v. *muſtuckā.* مصطكي

(1183) عنب IN-UB. Grapes. *vide* 885.

(1184) عنب الثعلب IN-UB US SÁ-LEB. Fox's grapes, nightſhade.

मकोय *má-ko-ey.*

p. *robá tirbuc.* روباه تربك

    prop. repellent. *ch.* yellow, and freſh. *cor.* ſugarcandy, or honey.

(1185) عناب UN-ÁB. Jujubes.

    prop. emollient. *d.* in decoction fifteen plùms. *ſuc.* raiſins.

(1186) عنكبوت UN-KE-BOOT. A ſpider. मकरी h. *muckree.*

p. *de-yú-pa.* دیوپا

(1187) عنزروت UNZEROOT. Sarcocolla. *vide* 290.

(1188) عنبر UMBIR. Ambergris.

    prop. cephalic, and cardiac. *ch.* of an aſh colour.

(1189) عنصل UNSOOL. Squills. *vide* 139.

(1190) عندم UNDUM. Red ſaunders. p. *buckum.* بقم

(1191) عود الصليب OWD US SE-LEEB. Name of a root. *vide* 1203.

(1192) عود العطاس OWD-UL-UT-ÁS. ſneezewort. *vide* 209.

(1193) عود الدرقه OWD-UD-DER-KEH. Root of the aſafœtida plant.

p. *beikh ungudán.* بیخ انكدان

(1194) عود هندي OWD HINDEE. Lignum aloes. *vide*

    prop. deobſtruent, diaphoretic, cephalic, and cardiac. *d.* half a direm.

(1195) عین ÁIN. An eye.

आंख h. *ánkh.*   p. *cheſhem.* چشم

        C c   (1196)

غ

(١١٩٦) غافث GHÁFIS. Hemp-agrimony.

prop. deobftruent   *ch.* Perfian.   *d.* one mifkal.

(١١٩٧) غار GHAR.   The laurel.

prop. difcutient and attenuant.   *d.* half a mifkal.

(١١٩٨) غاسول GHÁSOOL.   Glaff-wort. *vide* 163.

(١٢٩٩) غاربغون GHA-REE-KOON.   Agaric.

prop. deobftruent; deftroying worms; cathartic. *d.* one or two dangs.   *fuc.* as a cathartic turbeth root; and wormfeed againft worms.

(١٢٠٠) غرب GHIRB.   The mountain pine.

prop. drying.   *ch.* the fruit.

(١٢٠١) غورة GHOWREH.   Every kind of green fruit.

ف

(١٢٠٢) فاشرا FÁSHERA.   Bryony.

p. kerm defhty. كرمدشتي

(١٢٠٣) فاوانيا FÁ-WE-NYÁ.   A root.

p. owd felub. عودصليب

prop. aftringent, deobftruent, and diaphoretic. *d.* half a mifkal.   *cor.* tragacanth.   *fuc.* agaric, and round birthwort.

(١٢٠٤) فادج FÁDUJ.   Bezoar ftone.

जहरमोहरः *h. zehr mohrd.*   *p. pádzir kánee.* پادزهركاني

(١٢٠٥) فانيذ FÁ-NEEZ.   A kind of barley fugar. वताहः *h. be-tá-feh.*

(١٢٠٦) فار FÁR.   A rat, or moufe.

चुहा *h. chewhá.*   *p. moofh.* موش

(١٢٠٧) فاخته FÁKHTEH.   A dove.

पेंडुकी *h. pindekee.*

(١٢٠٨) فجل FUJL.   A radifh.

मूली *h. moolee.*   *p. toorb.* ترب

(١٢٠٩) فرنجمشك FERENJ MISHK. A fpecies of fweet bafil. नौलसी *h. tulfee.* *p. bálungoo khoord.* بالنكوي خورد

(١٢١٠) فربيون FIR-BE-YOON, and فرفيون FIR-FE-YOON. Euphorbium.

P.

p. *sheer derukht zekoom.* شیر درخت زقوم

prop. cauſtic, attenuant, and cathartic. *ch.* yellow, and clean.

(1211) فراسیون FE-RÁ-SE-YOON. Wild leek.

p. *gund-ná-iy kouhee.* کند ناي کوهي

(1212) فستق FISTOOK. Piſtachio.

p. *piſteh.* پسته

(1213) فضه FIZZEH. Silver.

रुपा h. *roopa.* p. *nockeráh.* نقره

(1214) فطر FETR. Muſhroom.

p. *ſimaroogh.* سماروغ

(1215) فطراسالیون FETRA-SÁ-LI-YOON. Seed of wild parſley.

tokhem kerefs kouhee. تخم کرفس کوهي

(1216) فلفل اسود FILFIL USWUD. Black pepper.

मिर्च

h. *meeritch* p. *filfil ſee-áh.* فلفل سیاه

(1217) فلفل دراز FILFIL DRAJ. Long pepper. पिपलपिलू h. *pilpil.*

(1218) فلفل ابیض FILFIL Á-BI-YÚZ. White pepper.

filfil ſepeid. فلفل سپید

(1219) فلنج مشک FELUNJ MISHK. The ſame as No. 1209.

(1220) فل FUL. Root of the Indian nelufir.

p. *beikh nelufir hindee.* بیخ نیلوفر هندي

(1221) فلفل مویه FILFIL MOOYEH. Root of the long pepper buſh.

पीपलामूल h. *peeplámool.* p. *beikh derukht filfil dráz.* بیخ درخت فلفل دراز

(1222) فلفل بري FILFIL BIRREE. Seed of the agnus caſtus.

(1223) فنطافلون FEN-TA-FE-LOON. Cinquefoil.

p. *punjungooſht.* پنجنگشت

(1224) فوفل FOOFUL. Beetlenut.

सुपारी h. *soopáree.*

prop. aſtringent. *d.* half a direm.

(1225) فو FOO. Valerian.

जालनकरी h. *jal-láckree.*

prop. attenuant. *ch.* freſh, fragrant. *d.* half a direm. *ſuc.* aniſeed.

(1226) فوه FOOH. Madder.

ت

(1227) قاراسیا KERÁ SYÁ. Cherries. p. *áloo báloo.* آلوبالو

(1228) قاقله KÁKELEH. Cardamoms. *vide* 18.

(1229) قانصه KÁ-NI-SEH. The gizzard of any bird. पछरी h. *put hree.* p. *fungdáneh.* سنکدانه

(1230) قتاد KE-TÁD. The tree which produces gum tragacanth. p. *kum.* کم

(1231) قثا KE-SÁ. A fpecies of long cucumber. ककूरी h. *kuckree.* p. *khyár dráz.* خیاردراز

(1232) قثاءالحمار KE-SÁ-UL HY-MÁR. Wild cucumber. करेला h. *kereylá.*

  prop. cathartic and emetic. *d.* of the expreffed juice two dáneks. *cor.* tragacanth.

(1233) قت KE-TÁH. A fpecies of clover. v. *ifpifs.* اسپست

(1234) قردمانا KOOR-DU-MÁ-NÁ. Cardmine.

  v. *kur-we-yá jebulee.* کرویاجبلي

  prop. deobftruent, attenuant, and diaphoretic. *d.* one mifkal. *cor.* anifeed. *fuc.* muftard feed.

(1235) قرن البحر KERN-UL-BEHR.

Amber. p. *kehro-bá.* کهربا

(1236) قرمز KERMEZ. Kermes, ufed in dying.

(1237) قرع KE-RÁ. A fpecies of gourd. p. *kud-oo.* کدو

(1238) قرنفل KERUNFUL. Cloves. लौंग h. *lowng.* p. *meykuc.* میخک

(1239) قرون السنبل KEROON US SEMBEL. A poifonous plant, the filaments of which are fometimes found amongft Indian fpikenard. संगियाजहर h. *fun-gee-yá-zehr.*

(1240) قرفةالقرنفل KERFET'UL KERUNFUL. An aromatic bark, of the colour of cloves.

(1241) قرن KERN. Horn. सींग h. *feeng.* p. *fhákh.* شاخ

(1242) قرطم KOORTEM. Safflower. *vide* 44-450-856.

(1243) قرةالعین KOORUT'L AIN. A kind of water creffes. p. *kerefs ul máá.* کرفس الما

  prop. detergent; and deftroying worms. *d.* in decoction five direms.

(1244)

(1244) قرطم هندي KOORTEM HINDEE. A purgative feed.

v. hub ul neel. حب النيل

(1245) قسط KUST. Coſtus.

(1246) قسطاهندي KUST-HINDEE. Bitter coſtus. p. kuſt telkh. قسطاتلخ

(1247) قشر KISHR. Bark of any tree. चल्का h. chilká. p. poſt. پوست

(1248) قصببوا KUSSEB BEWÁ. Calamus aromaticus. vide 672.

(1249) قصب KUSSEB. The common reed. p. nie. ني

(1250) قصب السكر KUSSEB U'S SOOKIR. Sugar cane. h. ऊख ookh. p. nie ſhuckir. نيشكر

(1251) قطونا KUT-OO-NÁ. Fleawort. p. uſ-pe-ghool. اسپغول

(1252) قطن KOOTN. Cotton. रूई h. rewie. p. pembeh. پنبه

(1253) قطران KIT-RÁN. Pitch.

(1254) قلت KOOLT. Saxifrage. v. kaſir ul hejr. كاسرالحجر

(1255) قلب KULB. The heart p. dil. دل

(1256) قلي KIL-EE. Soap aſhes. साजी h. ſajee. v. kil-ee-yá قليا

(1257) قنب KINNUB. Hemp. भांग h. bángh. p. báng. بنك prop. narcotic, and inebriating.

(1258) قيل KEEL. Pitch. राल h. rál. p. keer. قير

(1259) قيصوم KYSOOM. Mugwort. v. bir-un-já ſif. برنجاسف

ک

(1260) كاهربا KÁH-RO-BÁ. Amber.

(1261) كاكنج KÁKE-NUJ. Winter cherry. vide 443.
prop. narcotic. d. two direms.

(1262) كافور KÁ-FOOR. Camphor.

(1263) كاجر GÁ-JIR. गाजर Carrot.

(1264) كاشم KÁ-SHEM. The aſafœtida plant.

D d

(1265)

(1265) كاوزبان GÁO-ZEBÁN. p. Buglofs. a. *liffán us faur.* لسان‌الثور

(1266) كاهو KÁ-HOO. Lettuce. p. *khufs.* خس

(1267) كاسني KÁ-SE-NEE. कासनी Endive. p. *hin-de-bá.* هندبا

(1268) كانكني KÁN-GNEE. कांगनी Millet. p. *urzun.* ارزن

(1269) كبريت KIB-REET. Sulphur. गंधक h. *gundhuck.* p. *gowgird.* كوكرد *prop* attenuant, and drying. *d.* as far as two direms. *cor.* water melon.

(1270) كبيكج KUB-EE-KUJ. Water crefses. देवकांदुर h. *deo-kán-dur.*

(1271) كبر KUB-IR. Capers.

(1272) كپاس KÉ-PASS. कपास The cotton fhrub.

p. *derukht pembeh.* درخت‌پنبه

(1273) كبابه KE-BÁ-BEH. Cubebs.

(1274) كنك KUT-UC. The crab apple. p. *feeb birree.* سيب‌بري

(1275) كنهل KUT-HUL. कटहल An Indian fruit, called by Europeans, *jack,* and which refembles the hedgehog.

(1276) كتان KUT-ÁN. Linfeed. p. *ulfee.* السي

(1277) كثيرا KE-SEE-RÁ. Gum tragacanth. कटीरा h. *kuthee-rá.* *prop.* allaying thirft. *d.* half a mifkal. *cor.* anifeed. *fuc.* gum arabic.

(1278) كچور KE-CHOOR. कचुर Zerumbád. p. *zerumbád.* زرنباد

(1279) كچنار KUTCH-NÁR. कछनार An Indian tree, bearing purple buds, which the natives boil and eat with bread or rice.

(1280) كجپيپل GUJ-PEEPUL. गजपीपल् The fruit of the *cháb* tree. p. *femr cháb.* ثمرچاب

(1281) كچلون KUTCHLOON. कछनोन् The drofs of glafs.

p. *nim-uck fheefheh.* نمك‌شيشه

(1282) كحل ROHUL. Antimony. ऄंजं h. *unjen.* p. *foormeh.* سرمه

(1283) كدوي‌تلخ KUD-EW-EE TELKH. *p.* The bitter gourd. तोंबरी h. *toombree.*

(1284) كدم KUD-UM. कदंमू An Indian yellow flower, round like a ball.

(1285)

(1285) كرويا KUR-WEE-YÁ. Caraway seed.

(1286) كروندا KEROWNDÁ. करौंदा An Indian fruit, refembling the goofeberry.

(1287) كرنب KIR-NUB. Cabbage. p. *ke-lum.* كلم prop. emollient, and fuppurative.

(1288) كراث KOORNÁSS. Leeks. *gun-de-ná.* كندنا

(1289) كرفس KEREFS. Parfley. अजमूद h. *ujmood.* prop. deobftruent, and diaphoretic. *ch.* garden.

(1290) كرش KOORSH. Tripe. उजरी h. *uj-e-ree.* v. *fhe-kum-beh.* شكنبه

(1291) كرگ KIRG. The rhinoceros. गैंडा h. *gyndá.* p. *kur-gud-án.* كركدن

(1292) كرگ GOORG. *p.* The wolf. हुनडार h. *hoondár.*

(1293) كرم KERM. The vine. *vide* 194.

(1294) كركم KOORKUM. Saffron.

(1295) كزمازک GUZ-MA-ZUC. The fruit of the tamarifk tree.

(1296) كزانكبين GUZ-UNGU-BEEN. A fpecies of manna collected from the tamarifk tree.

(1297) كسير KU-SEER. Dry pitch. p. *zift kooßhk.* زفتخشك

(1298) كسنبه KU-SUMBH. कुसुंभ Safflower. *vide* 450. v. *másfir.* معصفر

(1299) كستوري KUS-TOO-REE. Mufk. p. *mooßhk.* مشك

(1300) كشمش KISHMISH. A fpecies of raifins without feed. v. *me-weez ungoor beydáneh.* مویزانكوربیدانه

(1301) كشوثرومي KU-SHOOS ROOMEE. Wormwood. *vide* 224.

(1302) كل GOOL. *p.* Any flower. फुल्ल h. *phool.*

(1303) كل GIL. *p.* Earth, clay.

(1304) كلاغ KE-LÁGH. *p.* A crow. v. *zág.* زاغ a. *gherab.* غراب कौवा h. *kow-wá.*

(1305) كلم KE-LUM. *p.* A cabbage.

(1306) كليجن KO-LEE-JUN. Galangal. *vide* 855.

(1307)

(1307) كانيطوس KE-MÁ-FEE-TOOS. Ground pine.

p. *máshdároo.* ماشداروو

prop. deobstruent, and detergent. *d.* one miskal. *cor.* aniseed.

(1308) كمادريوس KE-MÁ-DREE-YOOS. Germander.

prop. attenuant, deobstruent, and diaphoretic. *d.* one miskal. *cor.* quince. *suc.* agrimony.

(1309) كمرك KUMRUCK. कंरकू An Indian fruit.

(1310) كمون KE-MOON. Cumin feed. जी रा: h. *zeeráh.*

(1311) كمثري KU-MUS-RÁ. *a.* A pear, *vide* 274.

prop. astringent, and cardiac. *d.* of the juice one wekyáh. *cor.* honey and water. *suc.* quinces.

(1312) كنار KÓ-NÁR. A species of plum. बोर h. *be-ir.*

(1313) كندر KOONDIR. Frankincense.

prop. narcotic. astringent, styptic, cephalic, and cardiac. *ch.* white round grains. *d.* half a direm. *suc.* mastich.

(1314) كنير KE-NEER. इनेर Rhododaphne. p. *khurzereh.* خرزهره

(1315) كهربا KEH-RO-BA. Amber.

(1316) كهار KHAR. ख़ार Salt obtained from burnt vegetables; fixed alkaline salt.

(1317) كهيوكوار GHEEKWAR. घीकिवार The aloe plant.

(1318) كهاريلون KÁ-REE-LOON. गारिलोनू Sea salt.

p. *nemuck shoor.* نمكشور

(1319) كهنكي GHOONG-CHEE. घोंगत्री A red berry used as a weight, and commonly called a *rutty.* *vide* 759.

(1320) كيلا KAY-LA. केला The plantain, the Indian fig. v. *mowz.* موز

(1321) كيسر KEY-SIR. Saffron.

(1322) كيل KEEL. *p.* The medlar. *vide* 622. v. *zá-roos.* زعرور

(1323) كيسو KEY-SOO. An odoriferous grass.

ل

ل
___

(1324) لاژورد LAZJÉ-WIRD. Lapis lazùli.   v. *lajwird*.   لاجورد

prop. cathartic and cardiac. *ch.* Budakhſhany.
d. one direm. *cor.* maſtich.

(1325) لادن LÁ-DUN. Labdanum,
a reſinous ſubſtance.

prop. attenuant, ſuppurative, diſcutient. *ch.*
greaſy, of a yellow tinge. *d.* one direm. *cor.*
roſe water and ſandal wood.

(1326) لاغيه LÁ-GHEEYETT. A milky plant, bearing a yellow flower, and
whoſe leaves are tinged with the ſame
colour. It grows at the foot of mountains..

prop. cauſtic. *ch.* very juicy.   *d.* two dangs..
cor. tragacanth.

(1327) لاكه LAKH. लाग Stick lac.
v. *look*.   لكك

(1328) لبلاب LUBLAB. Ivy.
v. *aiſhk peitchán*.   عشق پیچان

(1329) لبن LEBN. Milk.
द्ध h. *dood*.   p. *ſheir*. شیر

(1330) لبان LUBÁN. Olibanum, a
ſpecies of frankincenſe.
v. *koondir*.   كندر

(1331) لحم LEHM. Fleſh.

माम h. *máſs*.   p. *gowſht*. كوشت

(1332) لحيةالتيس LEHEET-ÚT
TEES. Goat's beard, a ſhrub.
p. *derukht ſeers*.   درخت سرس

prop. aſtringent.   *d.* one miſkal to two direms.
cor. aniſeed.

(1333) لسان الكلب LISSÁN UL
KULB. Hound's tongue ; cynogloſſum.

(1334) لسان لثور LISSÁN U'S SAUR.
Bugloſs. *vide* 6-68.

(1335) لسان الحمل LISSÁN UL
HEML. Arnogloſſum.
p. *weruck bártung*.   ورق بارتنک

(1336) لعبت بربري LÁ-BUT BIR-
BIRREE. Hermodactyls. *vide* 179-797.

(1337) لغاح LU-FÁH. Fruit of the
mandrake.

(1338) لوبيا LOO-BEE-YÁ. A ſpecies of bean.

prop. diaphoretic, and emetic. *ch.* red.

(1339) لوزحلووُمِر LOUZ HELOU
WU MURR. Sweet and bitter almonds.   p. *bá-dam*

ſheer

shereen wu telkh. بادام شیریں و تلخ

prop. The sweet, provocative, and the bitter, deobstruent. *ch.* large and oily. *d.* ten direms.

(1340) لوطوس LOOTOOS. Syr.
The lotus, or water lily.

कंवल h. *kowul.*

a. *hundkookee.* حندقوقي

p. *neelufir.* نیلوفر

(1341) لوف LOOF. Dragonwort.
vide 67-183.

prop. destroying worms; deobstruent. *d.* one direm. *cor.* endive. *suc.* root of the caper bush.

(1342) لوبان LOOBAN. Male frankincense, of a reddish tinge.

v. *koondir zuckir.* كندرذكر

(1343) لولو LOOLOO. Pearl.

मोती h. *mow-tee.*

p. *mir-wár-reed.* مروارید

(1344) لیلنج LEE-LUNJ. The Indigo plant. v. *neel.* نیل

(1345) لیمو LEE-MOO. A lemon.
नेंबू h. *neem-boo.*

م

(1346) مامیثا MÁ-MEE-SÁ. A species of poppy.

(1347) مارماهیج MAR-MÁ-HEEJ.
The eel. बाममछली h. *bam mutchlee.*
p. *mar-má-hee.* مارماهي

(1348) ماءالشعیر MÁ-U'S-SHI-EER.
Barley water.

जौपानी h. *jow pá-nee.*

(1349) ماش MASH. A species of pea.
मोंग h. *mowng* p. *be-noo-másh.* بنوماش

(1350) مازریون MÁ-ZIR-YOON.

Mezereon root. p. *mustroo.* مستِ رو

prop. detergent, and cathartic; the seed emetic. *ch.* the plant full of leaves. *d.* half a direm. *cor.* steeping it in vinegar.

(1351) مامیران MÁ-MEE-RÁN.
A species of yellow wood.
prop. deobstruent, and diaphoretic.

(1352) ماهفرفین MAH-FIR-FEEN.
Zedoary. p. *judwár.* جدوار

(1353) مارچوبه MAR-CHOO-BEH.
Asparagus. नाकदौन h. *nákdown.*
v. *hil-*

v. *hil-yoon.* هليون p. *márgee-ah.* مارکیاه

(1354) مازو MAZOO. Gall apple.

माजुफलू h. *má-joo-phul.* p. *uf-is.* عفص

(1355) ماهودانه MÁHOO-DÁNEH.

माहुदाना A feed.

v. *hub ul mullook.* حب الملوک

    prop. emetic, and cathartic. *d.* one direm.

(1356) ماش هندي MÁSH HINDEE.

p. Saxifrage.

पंवाल h. *punwar.* v. *koolt.* قلت

(1357) منثر MUT̤HUR. मठर Peas.

p. kir-se-neh. کرسنه

(1358) مثلث MU'-SUL-US. Juice

of grapes boiled down to one third.

(1359) مثنان MUS-NÁN. A fpecies

of mezereon, which produces the feed

called *kirm dá-neh.*

(1360) مجنج MOOJ-NUJ. A plant

whofe leaves are beautifully variegated.

कुलफा h. *kulfa.* p. *khooshnuz-ir.* خوش نظر

(1361) مجينه ME-JEET̤H. मजीठ:

Red wood. *a. buckum.* بقم

(1362) محلب MELUB. A tree bear-

ing a berry called *hub mehlub,* and

which refembles pear feed.

(1363) محروث MEH-ROOS. Roo

of the afafœtida plant.

    prop. attenuant. *ch.* white, and light.

(1364) مرقشيشا MIR-KÁ-SHEE-SHA.

Marcafite. *vide* 82.

सोमाजी h. *foon-mukhee.*

v. *hejr ulnoor.* حجرالنور

    prop. aftringent.

(1365) مرماحوز MIRMÁ-HOOZ.

A fpecies of merow. *vide* 1375.

(1366) مروشك MIR-WIRUSHK.

A fpecies of merow. *vide* 1375.

(1367) مردارسنج MOORDÁRSUNJ.

Litharge of lead.

p. moordar-fung. مردارسنک

(1368) مر MURR. Myrrh.

बोल h. *bowl.*

(1369) مرمر MIRMIR. Marble.

(1370) مرزنجوش MIR-ZUN-

JOASH. Marjoram.

(1371) مرق MÉ-RUCK. Broth.

p. fhoorbá. شوربا

(1372) مرجان MER-JÁN.

Coral. *vide* 417-484-781.

(1373) مراينيه ME-RÁ-NEE-YEH.

A

A tree refembling jafmin. There are two fpecies; that which is moft fragrant, or *mirmáhooz*; and another lefs fragrant, called *femoofeh* and *mirwirufhk*. *vide* 1357 and 1368.

(1374) مزمارالراعي MIZMAR UR RÁIY. Shepherd's pipe; called alfo fhepherd's ftaff. *vide* 61.

(1375) مس MISS. *p.* Copper. तांबा h. *tambá.* a. *noháʃ.* نحاس

(1376) مسك MISK. Mufk. *vide* 1299. कस्तूरी h. *kuftowree.* p. *mooʃhk.* مشك

(1377) مشمش MISHMISH. Apricot. खुबानी h. *khoobánee.* p. *zirdáloo.* زردآلو

(1378) مشكالرمان MISHK UR' RÁ MÁN. A beautiful flower tree. नागेसर h. *nágeyfir.*

(1379) مصطكي MUSTEKÁ Maftich.

(1380) معصفر MÁSFIR. Safflower. *vide* 44-456-966.

(1381) مغرة MOGHRAH. Red earth.

prop. aftringent; drying. *ch.* bright red. *d.* half a mifkal. *cor.* honey.

(1382) مغناطيس MIK-NÁ-TEES. The magnet.

चमकूपहर h. *chum-uck puther.* p. *fung áhun robá.* سنك اهن ربا

(1383) مقل MOKUL. Bdellium. *vide* 222-408-864-908.

(1384) ملح MELH. Salt. नोन h. *loon.* p. *nemuck.* نمك

(1385) ملخ MUL-UC. A Locuft. टिड्डी h. *tidde e.* a. v. *jé-rád.* جراد

(1386) من MUNN. Manna; general name for all kinds of honey dew. *vide* 611.

(1387) موي كياه MOO-EY GEE-AH. The hairy grafs; Indian fpikenard. *vide* 150-724-726.

(1388) مورد MOWRID. Myrtle. *vide* 127. v. *áfs.* آس

(1389) موز MOWZ. The plantain, or Indian fig. h. *key-lá.* केला

(1390) موته MOWTH. A fmall Indian grain. मोठ:

(1391) موميايي MO-MEE-IY. Mummy.

(1392) مهاور MEHÁ-WIR. Tincture of gum lac.

(1393)

(1393) می MEY. *p.* Wine.

मद h. *mud.* *a. khumr.* خمر

(1394) میندهاسینکي MEYNDEH SINGEE. An Indian milky plant.

ن

(1395) ناخن بویا NÁKHUN BÚ-YÁ. Perfumed nails. *vide* 208.

नरव h. *nukh.*

(1396) نارنج NÁ-RUNJ. An orange.

(1397) نارجیل NÁR-JEEL. A cocoanut. *vide* 722.

(1398) ناردین NARDEEN. Celtic nard. *v. sembel roomee.* سنبل رومي

(1399) ناکدون NÁKDOWN. Asparagus. *vide* 1437.

(1400) ناخن دیو NAKHUN-DEO. Perfumed nails. *vide* 1395.

(1401) نانخواه NÁN-KHAH. A species of aniseed.

(1402) نحل NEHL. A bee. p. *mug-us á-sul.* مكس عسل

(1403) نخل NUKHEL. The date or palm tree.

p. *derukht khurmá.* درخت خرما

(1404) نخاله NE-KHÁ-LEH. Chaff.

मुसी h. *bhoosee.* · p. *se-boos.* سبوس

(1405) نرجس NUR-JISS. The narciffus. p. *nurgis.* نرکس

(1406) نسرین NUSSREEN. The China rofe; the dog-rofe. सेवती h. *sow-tee* v. *wurd cheenee.* ورد چیني

(1407) نشاسته NE-SHÁS-TEH. *p.* Starch.

a. *lubáb ul kum-eh.* لباب القمح

(1408) نطرون NUTROON. A fpecies of borax. जवाखार h. *jewakhar.* p. *booreh urmenee.* بوره ارمني

(1409) نعنع NÁ-NÁ. *a.* Mint. *vide* 559.

(1410) نغط NEFT. *a.* Bitumen.

(1411) نمل NEML. *a.* An ant. चींवटी h. *choontee.* p. *moorcháh.* مورچه

(1412) نمام NE-MAM. Mother of thyme. बिरनान h. *bir-nán.* v. *see-sum-bir.* سیسنبر

Ff (1413)

(1413) نیلج NEE-LUJ. Indigo. v. uſſáreh neel. عصارة نیل p. neeleh. نیله

(1414) نیلوفر NEELUFIR. The winter lily. कॉंवल h. kenowl.

(1415) نیل NEEL. The Indigo plant.

(1416) نیپال NY-PAL. नैपाल A ſpecies of wormſeed plant.

و

(1417) وج WUJ. Sweet ſcented flag. बच h. butch. p. ug-ir toor-kee. اکر ترکي

(1418) ورد WURD. a. The red roſe. p. gul. گل

(1419) ورددفلي WURD DIFLEE. The rhododaphne roſe.

कनेकीफूल h. káneer-kd-phool.

(1420) وسمه WUS-MEH. A plant, of which women make a decoction, for dying the eyebrows black.

p. weruck neel. ورق نیل

و

(1421) هدلزنكي HU-DUL ZUN-GEE. Turbith root.

निसबतू h. nys-wul.

(1422) هرتال HURTAL. हरताल Yellow orpiment. v. zirneekh zird. زرنیخ زرد

(1423) هلیلج HE-LEE-LUJ. Yellow myrobalans. हरड h. hirra.

(1424) هلدي HULDEE. हलदी Turmeric. v. zird-choobeh. زردچوبه

(1425) هلیون HULYOON. Aſparagus.

prop deobſtruent, and diaphoretic. ch. garden. d. of the ſeed two direms.

(1426) هندبا HIN-DU-BA. Endive. p. káſnee. کاسني

(1427) هیلبوا HEEL BU-YA. The leſſer cardamom ſeed. v. ká-keleh ſe-ghár. قاقلهصغار

(1428) هینك HINGH. हींग Aſafœtida. vide 305-798.

(1429) هیضبان HE-ZEE-MAN. Horſe raddiſh. p. toorb birree. ترسبري ي

ي

(1430) ياقوت YE-Á-COOT. A ruby.

(1431.) ياسمين YE-ÁS-MEEN.
Jaſmin. चंबेली h. *chumbeylee.*
prop. the flowers attenuant, and cephalic. *ch.*
white, fragrant. *cor.* camphor.

(1432) يبروج YEB-ROOJ. Mandrake.
vide 137-173-621.

(1433) ينوع YE-TUÁ. A general
name for all milky plants.

(1434) يخصص YUKH-SIS. A ſpecies
of parſley, larger than the common
plant.

(1435) يخچه YEKH-CHEH. *p.*
Hailſtones. ओला h. *owlá. p. te-gurg,*
and *zhá-leh.* ژاله تکرک

(1436) يذنقه YUZ-KEH. *v.* The
dwarf elder.
v. khámá'uktee. حاماءاقطي

(1437) يراميع YE-RÁ-MY-Á. *a.*
aſparagus. *vide* 1400.

(1438) يشف YESHF. Jaſper.
p. ſung ye-ſhem. سنك يشم

(1439) يقطين YUKTEEN. *a.* A
general name for plants having tendrils.

(1440) يلنجوج YE-LUN-JOOJ.
Lignum aloes. *p. oud hindee.* عود هندي

(1441) ينبوت YUMBOOT. A ſpecies of bean.
p. khirnub nubtee. خرنوب نبطي

www.ingramcontent.com/pod-product-compliance
Ingram Content Group UK Ltd.
Pitfield, Milton Keynes, MK11 3LW, UK
UKHW050103180125
453697UK00022B/519